Child safety: problem and prevention from preschool to adolescence

Child safety is everyone's concern, but who bears responsibility for it, and are we prepared to pay for it?

Written and edited by leading researchers into child safety, this book highlights the growing gap between current research findings, national policy and popular knowledge. This book points out the inherent weaknesses of *educational* approaches to the problem of child safety: the disturbing message is that simply improving our children's knowledge has little or no effect on their behaviour.

By challenging traditional approaches to child safety training, this comprehensive handbook presents a refreshingly new perspective on a key social issue. It also indicates approaches that are more likely to be effective in alleviating the problems of children's safety.

Dealing in depth with a wide range of topics, from physical abuse of young children to drug abuse in adolescence, this collection is essential for all those with an interest in child welfare.

Bill Gillham is Senior Lecturer in the Department of Psychology at the University of Strathclyde, and is the author of numerous publications on the prevention of physical and sexual child abuse. He has also written a wide variety of books for children. **James A. Thomson** is Reader in Psychology at the University of Strathclyde and has published extensively on the psychology of children's accidents. He is currently involved in developing more effective road safety education schemes.

Child safety: problem and prevention from preschool to adolescence

A handbook for professionals

Edited by Bill Gillham and
James A. Thomson

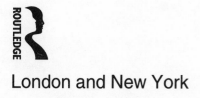

London and New York

First published 1996
by Routledge
11 New Fetter Lane, London EC4P 4EE

Simultaneously published in the USA and Canada
by Routledge
29 West 35th Street, New York, NY 10001

Typeset in Palatino by LaserScript, Mitcham, Surrey
Printed and bound in Great Britain by
TJ Press (Padstow) Ltd, Padstow, Cornwall

British Library Cataloguing in Publication Data
A catalogue record for this book is available from the British Library

Library of Congress Cataloguing in Publication Data
A catalogue record for this book has been requested

ISBN 0–415–12476–X (hbk)
ISBN 0–415–12477–8 (pbk)

Contents

Figures

Tables

Contributors

Bill Gillham is Senior Lecturer in the Department of Psychology at Strathclyde University. He is currently researching the epidemiology of child abuse in Glasgow and Strathclyde, a project funded by the Nuffield Foundation. He is the author of two books on child sexual abuse and physical abuse, has published a number of papers and has written television programmes for children dealing with sexual abuse prevention.

James A. Thomson is Reader in the Department of Psychology at Strathclyde University. He is the author of a book and numerous scientific papers on the psychology of children's road accidents. He is currently director of two major research programmes aimed at developing more effective road safety education schemes through the application of psychological principles. In 1994 he was commissioned with Andrew Tolmie and Hugh Foot to write a major critical review of road safety education, for the Department of Transport, which will shortly be published by HMSO. This review has led to the Child Development Research Programme, a government-funded research initiative aimed at increasing our understanding of the psychological factors underlying child pedestrian accidents.

Helen Roberts works as a mother and as Co-ordinator of Research and Development at Barnardo's. She was involved in a number of child accident initiatives in Glasgow, and has a longstanding interest in inequalities in maternal and child health. Her publications include *Doing Feminist Research*, *Women's Health Matters* and *Women's Health Counts*. Her most recent book, written with Susan J. Smith and Carol Bryce is *Children at Risk? Safety as a Social Value*.

David Warden is Senior Lecturer in the Department of Psychology at Strathclyde University, and works in the Centre for Research into Interactive Learning. He has directed a series of ESRC-funded research programmes concerned with children's safety, and is currently working on two projects: examining children's understanding of secrecy; and developing peer interaction methods for fostering prosocial behaviours and inhibiting antisocial behaviours amongst children.

James Boyle is Senior Lecturer and Director of the M.Sc. Educational Psychology course at Strathclyde University. Formerly a practising educational psychologist, he has a longstanding interest in the problems of bullying.

John B. Davies is Professor of Psychology at Strathclyde University. He has carried out centrally funded research into a number of aspects of addiction including drugs, alcohol and violence, drug use in prisons, the impact of alcohol and drugs in the workplace, and theories of addiction. He is currently involved in a World Health Organisation study into the effects of alcohol at work. He has published widely on the topic of addiction in academic journals. He is the author of a controversial book *The Myth of Addiction* and editor of the international journal *Addiction Research*.

Preface

We have learnt a lot in the editing of this book. All researchers are specialists, and reading the chapters of other contributors has clarified our thinking about topics outside our own specialisms of child abuse and child pedestrian accidents. This has supported our belief in the value of the book, and also in the value of research.

Individuals do research for many reasons. The intellectual challenge of making sense of an area of knowledge that is complex and significant is an obvious component. But all the researchers who have contributed to this book are also committed to making society a safer and more secure place for children to grow up in. Translating such a pious (and un-contentious) aim into practice is not easy. The difficulties are not just the technical problems of doing research, but the gap between current research, government policy, professional practice and popular knowledge. The present book, aimed at a wide audience, is an attempt partly to fill that gap. On its own it is a small contribution: the editors are under no illusions about that. But we see the consistent promotion of important research findings and their interpretation as essential, if social policy and social action are to be properly informed.

BG, JT
Department of Psychology, Strathclyde University

Acknowledgements

The main acknowledgement has to be to Anne Toland who standardised the word-processing of individual chapters to the same conventions. Judith Gillham read each chapter and significantly improved the level of writing in all of them.

We are grateful to The Open University Press and the Office of Population Censuses and Surveys for permission to reproduce copyright figures from Woodroffe, C., Glickman, M., Barker, M. and Power, C. (1993) 'Children, teenagers and health: the key data', Milton Keynes: Open University Press; Carfax Publishing Company for permission to reproduce a copyright table from Swadi, H. (1988) 'Drug and substance abuse among 3,333 London adolescents', *British Journal of Addiction* 83: 935–42; S. J. Creighton and the NSPCC for permission to reproduce copyright figures and a table from S. J. Creighton (1992) *Child Abuse Trends in England and Wales 1988–1990*, London: NSPCC; Professor David Lee and Elsevier Science Ltd for permission to reproduce a copyright figure from D. S. Young and D. N. Lee (1987) 'Training children in road crossing skills using a roadside simulation', *Accident Analysis and Prevention* 19, 5: 327–41; Professor David Lee and Messrs Taylor and Francis for permission to reproduce a copyright figure from D. N. Lee, D. S. Young and C. M. McLaughlin (1984) 'A roadside simulation of road crossing for children', *Ergonomics* 27, 12: 1271–81.

Chapter 1

The challenge of child safety research

Bill Gillham and James A. Thomson

Child safety is everyone's concern. The severe abuse, injury or death of a child brings about a public response of anger and outrage directed, not least, at those seen as responsible for protecting children. *Why weren't the police, social workers, teachers, etc. doing something about it?* This hindsight response to extreme cases implies that preventive action was obvious.

Indeed, when taken at face value, problems of child safety can seem largely a matter of common sense. But if so, why isn't it applied? The answer is that common sense at best over-simplifies the situation and is sometimes entirely wrong: and that if preventive measures are unsuccessful it is because the problem is complex and difficult to engage with. Professional workers often respond creatively but have to deal with a plethora of immediate demands that make it difficult to get beyond the current situation. The extra dimension provided by the research process is the time and space needed to reflect on issues, to get beyond immediacy, and to explore and evaluate new ways of dealing with the persistent problems of child safety.

DEFINING THE PROBLEM

Research can also help achieve a more balanced perspective. Because personal and even professional experience is restricted, it can often be biased. The picture gained from such experience is *real*, but it may not be *representative*. At one time, for example, it was thought that the sexual abuse of boys was much less common than the sexual abuse of girls – for the simple reason that most cases seen by doctors and social workers were of girls. Similarly, police officers may have good experience of road accidents involving child pedestrians but miss out on accidents that nearly happened, which may be an important part of the picture.

You cannot devise effective intervention and prevention procedures without an accurate view of the problem, a statement which may seem obvious until you start to examine the issues in depth. As we shall see, there is no entirely agreed view of the problem in relation to any of the topics discussed in this book. Contrary to what the cliché tells us, facts do not speak for themselves: they require qualification and interpretation. For example, it is in fact the case that as many mothers as fathers physically abuse children (at least according to the main UK study: Creighton, 1992). But in this study, it was found that children were twice as likely to be living with their mother as their father and therefore had far more contact with them. In other words, because the *exposure* was not equivalent, neither was the *risk*: fathers were more likely to abuse children when they were in contact with them.

The simple counting of numbers is not enough. To take another example, fewer children under five are killed on our roads than children over five. The risk is, nonetheless, greater for the younger children, but they are less *exposed to risk* in the first place. Another weakness of accident statistics is that they only reflect what happened – not what could have happened or nearly happened. In her chapters on accidents in the home Helen Roberts makes the important point that accident statistics tell us nothing about the strategies most parents use to keep their children safe most of the time. Without knowledge of 'near-misses' or the safety strategies that parents routinely adopt to protect their children, we may well see a distorted picture of what the problem is and how to solve it.

Most people, however, don't get their understanding of child safety issues from professional experience or from reading and studying the research literature which is, in any case, both extensive and diverse. For all of us, knowledge of those areas where we are not specialist comes largely through news reports and other media representations. News reports are written by journalists not by those with specialist experience, and it is not difficult to appreciate that correct facts may not be properly qualified or explained. But the problem is more than that. Media reports of child abuse and accidents are dominated by exceptional and dramatic cases: that is what makes them newsworthy. Such cases have an undeniable validity – they are terrible and they happened. But they do not adequately represent the problem: their extreme character is not characteristic.

News reports are one form of bias. Others are political, professional, and ideological. Bias from these sources is a complex issue and is considered more fully later under the heading 'Research and social policy'. Politicians' willingness to accept or consider research findings depends to some extent on whether the findings are likely to be acceptable to the electorate when translated into social policy; whether they are consistent with the beliefs of the relevant political party; and whether they would be troublesome to implement.

Something analogous happens in the reaction of relevant professionals. In the current climate, all professions are sensitive to evaluative research which might be seen to suggest their role is less crucial or effective than they would like. Professions too, have their ideologies. Whilst everyone wants to do the 'right thing' especially in relation to children and other vulnerable groups, what is seen as the right thing is going to be affected by its implications for professional practice, for social and political action, and to the extent that it aligns with beliefs or 'theories' that people hold. Systems don't change easily or quickly: it would be an unstable world if they did. Nor is there an implication here that the views of researchers should necessarily hold sway. They too have their preferred theories, though they approach them in a different way.

Professional (and other) 'resistance' to change is probably not the major problem. More problematic is that too much is almost certainly expected of practitioner professions – particularly social work and education. When evidence of greater social problems emerges, a common response from the public and politicians alike is to expect more of these overloaded professional groups or, indeed, to imply blame for their inaction. In relation to most social problems affecting school-age children, a common response is to impose further expectations on teachers. It is difficult to escape the inference that society shrugs off many of its responsibilities on to the teaching profession.

An assumption, usually tacit, is that an 'educational' response is what is needed to tackle the problem – be it sexual abuse, racial discrimination and harassment, or drug abuse. A great deal of money and energy is expended on developing programmes of this kind. But does a curriculum-based approach emphasising greater knowledge and changes in attitudes constitute effective intervention or prevention?

KNOWLEDGE ENHANCEMENT

A powerful and largely unquestioned assumption underlying almost all preventive approaches is that 'knowledge enhancement' is the way to deal with problems of personal safety. If children know what the risks are and are told what they should do to deal with them, then surely that will make them more safe? Unfortunately, a consistent finding is that such approaches do not work: increasing or improving children's knowledge certainly makes them better able to discuss the problems in the classroom and to give the 'right' answers when questioned by adults. But this increased knowledge does not generalise to their behaviour.

It is a paradox that at first seems surprising. After all, it is common sense that the difference between a novice and an expert is that the one knows more than the other. This view is naive, however, because expertise involves much more than 'knowing things': it implies being able to put that knowledge into practice. The difference between the master cabinet-maker and his apprentice is not that the master knows the steps to go through in cutting a dovetail joint, whereas the apprentice doesn't.

The difference is that the master *can do it*, whereas the apprentice can't (or does it much less well). The difference lies not so much in their *knowledge* as in their *skill*.

While probably much less apparent, the distinction between knowledge and skill holds true for the very different topics discussed in this book. In some cases, the analogy with the apprentice cabinet-maker may not seem too remote. For instance, learning how to cross the road safely involves specific skills like estimating vehicle distances and speeds. It is obvious that novice pedestrians, like novice cabinetmakers, would benefit from practical experience. But in the case of the more 'social' problems discussed in the book, the analogy may seem inappropriate.

However, such a view would be mistaken. For example, a major knowledge enhancement approach in trying to persuade young people not to dabble in drugs has been to inform them of how dangerous drugs are. There are several drawbacks to this approach. In the first place, it is not obvious that teenagers are particularly interested in avoiding dangerous activities: in fact, to be seen to do dangerous things can attract a great deal of esteem and kudos. For this reason, it may be much harder for the individual to refuse to participate than to join in. If the teenagers do intend to refuse, they may have to find a way of doing so without attracting the scorn of their peers. Just like cabinet-making this requires skill: in this case it is *social* skills that are required rather than physical ones. The same social skills are required in dealing with many of the situations discussed in this book: knowing how to reject unwelcome sexual advances, avoiding becoming the victim of bullying, all involve skill in dealing with the situations that arise in social contexts. There is thus little point in simply telling children and young people 'not to talk to strangers' or 'to say no to drugs': they need to learn how to deal with the concrete social encounters that arise in these contexts in an effective and skilled manner.

THE IMPORTANCE OF PRACTICAL TRAINING FOR CHILDREN

Knowledge enhancement, then, insofar as it simply informs children of risks or tells them verbally the general principles of how to cope, is of little help to them in dealing with a complex and sophisticated social and physical world. To do so effectively, they do not just need knowledge: they need 'know-how'.

By far the best way of getting know-how is through practical experience of dealing with appropriate situations, whether real or simulated. Obviously, these have to be modified so that no harm comes to children if they make errors. In learning how to deal with traffic situations, for instance, one can hardly set up training for children where they will make their mistakes crossing real roads. However, it is perfectly possible to contrive surrogates of real-life situations and use these as a tool for training. Just as apprentice pilots spend many hours in simulators developing their flying skills to the point at which they can begin to transfer them to real aircraft, so children would benefit from simulations that allow practical experience under equally controlled conditions. Later in the book we discuss how various simulations of the road environment can help to improve children's traffic judgements, sometimes quite dramatically. Similarly, role playing or other practical exercises might help children learn how to deal with some of the social situations that arise in the context of bullying, sexual advances from strangers and so on. The development of practical training methods to tackle such problems is very much in its infancy. For example, there is only one adequately evaluated sexual abuse prevention programme which has demonstrated *behavioural* generalisation (Fryer *et al.*, 1987); all others have judged success in terms of children's greater knowledge of what they should do. We argue that practical approaches aimed at improving children's behaviour rather than their knowledge deserve far greater emphasis than they have received up till now.

THE IMPORTANCE OF EVALUATION

It will be obvious, then, that not all preventive activities actually work in making children safer. Whether a particular programme does so is an empirical matter and requires demonstration. However, rigorous evaluation has seldom received a high priority in child safety research. As Thomson argues in his chapters on pedestrian safety, the attitude seems to be that if the material deals with child safety at all, then it is more or less bound to have a beneficial effect.

Most child safety programmes have enough 'face validity' to make evaluation appear almost unnecessary. The programme seems to make sense and is at least 'doing something about the problem', so what is there to complain about? However, quite a lot of things which at first sight seem to 'make sense' in fact don't work. Increasing children's knowledge may seem a good idea but if it doesn't lead to changes in how children behave in threatening situations, how much good has it actually done? Indeed, inappropriately formulated programmes may be positively harmful: for example, if parents feel that their children are now better equipped to deal with dangerous situations (e.g., the road environment) then they may allow them more access to roads in the mistaken belief that they are capable of handling them. In such a case, far from increasing the child's safety, the programme would positively increase the threat. It is therefore essential that programmes aimed at increasing children's safety should be evaluated with respect to their effectiveness, and realistic conclusions drawn as to what children can now do as a result of having undergone the programme (and, even more importantly, what they can't).

THE LIMITATIONS OF PREVENTIVE APPROACHES TARGETED ON CHILDREN

Helping children to behave more safely follows from the fact that adults cannot always be around to protect them. Eventually children must acquire the skills necessary to deal with life situations themselves. The question is whether they learn how to do so in a structured way through education, or whether they simply pick the skills up for themselves. Thomson argues in his chapters on road safety that this is precisely how most children learn to deal with traffic. If they survive they become quite good at it. Unfortunately, some become victims in the process. Nevertheless, it is important to assess as realistically as possible just what can be achieved through educational intervention and what can not. Many safety problems are intrinsically difficult for children and teaching them to cope with such situations may be a considerable challenge. For example, it is unlikely that any four-year-old could be taught road safety skills to a level that would enable them to become independent pedestrians. Road safety education for four-year-olds is essential, but the child is not being trained to become an independent pedestrian next week: they are being prepared for *future* independent travel. It is therefore incumbent on us to continue to protect the child for some years during which their training continues. Similarly, studies of child sexual abuse cases show that their predators are usually relatively sophisticated adults. Child molesters' accounts of how they identify and approach their victims make chilling reading (Budin and Johnson, 1989). Although children must learn to recognise and deal with such situations, there is a limit to their ability to do so. Two conclusions follow from this. Firstly, we need to know much more about what children of different ages are and are not capable of mastering in the context of child safety. Without such information, we cannot have a satisfactory basis for deciding what to teach to a particular age group or how to build on this as the child's experience changes. Secondly, educational initiatives must be matched by strenuous efforts to lower the risks posed by the physical and social environment in the first place.

Some approaches aimed at creating an intrinsically safer environment are elaborate and expensive, and cannot easily be introduced. An example would be the *woonerven* established in many Dutch cities. These are a sort of 'safe haven' in which pedestrians have (legally enforced) priority over vehicles and where the latter may travel only at very low speeds. In addition, such areas – which usually correspond to residential districts – are detached from main arterial roads so that there is no reason for vehicles to enter unless the driver lives in the area or is delivering goods or services. Such urban planning initiatives are effective but they are expensive and difficult to set up. It is unlikely that they will be introduced to any great extent in the UK.

However, it is surprising how effective relatively simple measures can be. For example, Hastings (1981) reported a reduction in playground bullying when he organised separately timed lunch breaks for older and younger pupils in his secondary school. This is simply because younger pupils are, as a group, the most vulnerable to bullying (see Chapter 10). Another relatively straightforward way of reducing risk, this time in the case of child sexual abuse, might be to further increase the thoroughness of vetting when adults apply for positions of responsibility towards children (molesters commonly seek such positions – see Chapter 9). The point is that measures can be taken to protect the child by making their world safer to begin with. Further efforts should be made to refine such techniques.

RESEARCH AND SOCIAL POLICY

Anyone with long experience of working in university social science departments cannot but be struck by the shift in research emphasis over the past twenty years. Research has become much more 'applied', more directly geared to social problems of one kind or another. This is certainly true in the case of psychology departments. Those who review large numbers of research grant applications are familiar with the 'relevance' claims for almost all of them, even when that claim is tenuous in the extreme.

Relevant or not, what researchers often lack is any conception of how research translates into social policy or becomes absorbed into the wider culture. What use is made of research (and is it used at all)? What is the role of the researchers themselves in the process? We can make a start to answering these questions by critically reviewing what we are doing ourselves.

The contributions to the present book demonstrate, over and over again, a 'rational' approach to the problems of child safety under review, i.e.

- arriving at a clear description and understanding of the problem;
- considering the effectiveness of different kinds of intervention and prevention.

What could be more obvious? As Lindblom observes: 'most people believe that the answer [to making policies more effective] lies in bringing more information, thought, and analysis into the policy-making process' (1980: 11).

Earlier we criticised 'knowledge enhancement' approaches to child safety (particularly when targetted on children). But such approaches have severe limitations when applied, for example, to health education targeted on adults. There can be few adult smokers who are not aware of the consequences of the habit for their future health; but knowing in that abstract way is not enough to change their behaviour.

There is an analogy here between the effect of rational knowledge enhancement approaches on individual behaviour, e.g. those who smoke, are overweight, etc. and the approach to complex social problems which require large-scale political and professional action. Researchers by the very 'rational' character of research activity can tacitly assume that increasing policy makers' 'knowledge' will influence their behaviour (i.e. their policy decisions). Bulmer (1986) points out:

> Those involved in knowledge production tend naturally to make assumptions about the rationality of the world and the advantages of having more knowledge rather than less. [It is suggested] that this is a wildly optimistic view of the process of social science influence, and that rational models of policy formation processes have a number of serious weaknesses. (1986: xviii)

The 'rationalist' assumptions of researchers, like the assumptions of health and safety educators, can underestimate the multiplicity of factors that lead to (or inhibit) change. This is true even of research that is explicitly set up by policy-makers. A form of social science research which is now quite common is where a government department directly commissions research in relation to a particular policy programme – the agenda being set by the politicians and administrators rather than the researchers, who are hired to 'do the job'.

Patricia Thomas of the Nuffield Foundation, one of the few in the UK to have systematically studied research utilisation concludes that 'the more closely . . . research is geared to policy, the less use will be made of it' (1987: 52). In part, this is because research proceeds slowly and policy priorities often change quickly; and largely because research findings are not, in a specific and immediate fashion, a major determinant of policy. She adds:

> Much of this lies unread in dusty corners of Whitehall . . . It will have signally failed to make a direct impact on policy-making because the parties involved in its inception – researcher, funding body and government department – too readily subscribed to the myth that research, by its very existence, can influence policy. (1987: 59)

Change, or reform, of any kind and whether fuelled by research or not, is a necessarily slow process. It requires a sustained policy (often not the case) and alterations, sometimes profound, to existing legislation, funding, public attitudes and professional practice. Researchers who expect a clear follow-through of the implications of their findings are not operating in the real world.

Fortunately most social scientists whose work may ultimately have a bearing on public policy and professional practice do not work in such a way or with such assumptions; if only because, to begin with at least, the implications of their research are not clear even to themselves. And, on the whole, researchers are cautious about such implications. Any student of the research literature (and with the benefit of hindsight) is struck by the latency of research findings: the relatively long period of time before they surface in the public consciousness and are formalised in policy and practice. It is as if the public mind has to be made receptive to new ideas that have been there in specialist circles for some time. Chapter 2 describes this process in relation to the 'battered child syndrome' first described in those terms in a paper by Kempe and his colleagues in 1962. The paper did little more than summarise a number of research studies from the previous twenty years, but the 1962 paper was the catalyst. Reading those earlier studies one can see that the authors were aware of professional resistance to their findings.

This particular example now seems obvious because we view it with hindsight. Emergent research is often troubling and uncomfortable. For example, recent research findings indicate that a proportion of so-called 'cot deaths' may be due to abuse (Emery, 1985; Southall et al., 1987; Newlands and Emery, 1991). Again there is much resistance to such findings and it will be some time before preferred explanations are modified, should the trend of the evidence persist.

Thomas (op. cit.) refers to the 'limestone model', a gradual process of influence to which she feels most policy research conforms. She comments:

> If social researchers had a monopoly on social comment, this limestone research would be extremely influential. But this is not the case. Journalists and broadcasters are also vying for the public's attention on the same or similar issues. Though social research may be more authoritative than a journalist's work, it may also be less accessible and less easily read. To say this is not to denigrate or in any way detract from the usefulness of limestone research, but there is more permeating the limestone than research. (1987: 58)

Bulmer (1986) makes a related point when he says: 'this is a messy, pluralistic world of negotiation and pressures of all kinds, into which social science feeds as one input among many. *This being so, the more widely the results of research can be disseminated the better*' (1986: xviii; emphasis added).

Such dissemination does not imply an expert-driven utopia where research findings achieve a direct translation into social action. Rather, it means ensuring that the results are exposed to political, professional and public *judgement*, as well as scrutiny by fellow researchers. In other words a research-driven appraisal of social problems is not enough. Changing policy or practice can have consequences far outside the scope or knowledge of the researcher. 'Resistance' to new findings may often be because change is not that simple.

The implication is not just that the wider world must be acquainted with research findings – important though that is – but that researchers have to understand better the ongoing social process which they seek to influence, and appreciate the practical and ethical problems of those actually implementing policy in their professional or other role.

All research has to be treated with caution: challenged, scrutinised, checked, replicated. Over-reaction to premature research findings can create more problems than it solves. For instance, at the time of writing there has been a scare about babies absorbing antimony vapour from flame-retardant mattresses and dying as a consequence. Further research has ruled this out as a possible cause of 'cot death'; but not before thousands of parents had replaced mattresses or lived in a state of heightened anxiety.

It is entirely right that the implications of research findings should be 'resisted' when the implications are profound; that researchers should have to justify themselves and be prepared to take into account the possible consequences (including negative effects) of what they are doing. Researchers have to make a distinction between working out the implications of their findings; and determining what exactly should be done in practice. The latter is not their province, except as partners in a process of negotiation. But if researchers have to take account of 'real world' practicalities, so do professionals and policy-makers have to work out the practical implications of, in particular, evaluative research: what doesn't work, and what might work. There is a tension here, but it can be a productive and healthy one. In the language of systems theory, systems that are too open to outside influences, that adapt too readily, become chaotic and unstable; systems that are too closed and seek to exclude outside influences which disturb their equilibrium, become increasingly ineffective. A balance has to be struck; and that applies to both practitioners and researchers.

REFERENCES

Budin, L. E. and Johnson, C. F. (1989) 'Sex abuse prevention programs: offenders' attitudes about their efficacy', *Child Abuse and Neglect* 13: 77–87.
Bulmer, M. (1986) 'Preface', in M. Bulmer (ed.) *Social Science and Social Policy*, London: Allen and Unwin.
Creighton, S. J. (1992) *Child Abuse Trends in England and Wales 1988–1990*, London: NSPCC.
Emery, J. L. (1985) 'Infanticide, filicide and cot death', *Archives of Disease in Childhood* 60: 505–7.
Fryer, G. E., Kraizer, S. K. and Miyoshi, T. (1987) 'Measuring actual reduction of risk to child abuse: a new approach', *Child Abuse and Neglect* 11: 173–9.
Hastings, J. (1981) 'One school's experience', in B. Gillham (ed.) *Problem Behaviour in the Secondary School*, London: Croom Helm.
Kempe, C. H., Silverman, F. N., Steele, B. F., Droegemuller, W. and Silver, H. K.

(1962) 'The battered-child syndrome', *Journal of the American Medical Association* 181, 1: 17–24.

Lindblom, C. (1980) *The Policy-Making Process* (2nd edition), Englewood Cliffs, NJ: Prentice-Hall.

Newlands, M. and Emery, J. L. (1991) 'Child abuse and cot deaths', *Child Abuse and Neglect* 15: 275–8.

Southall, D. P., Stebbens, V. A., Rees, S. V., Lang, M. H., Warner, J. O. and Shinebourne, E. A. (1987) 'Apnoeic episodes induced by smothering: two cases identified by covert video surveillance', *British Medical Journal* 294: 1637–41.

Thomas, P. (1987) 'The use of social research: myths and models', in M. Bulmer (ed.) *Social Science Research and Government*, Cambridge: Cambridge University Press.

Chapter 2

Physical abuse: the problem

Bill Gillham

What is physical abuse? Which is to ask: where is the boundary between legitimate and illegitimate violence towards children? By whom and in what contexts is it permissible to hit children? At the time of writing, the cases of a police officer and a child minder, who had slapped an adolescent and a preschool child respectively, have attracted a great deal of popular support and, in the end, a lenient official response.

Does a 'good slap' do children any harm? Probably not, but the point is that the ambiguity is there especially in relation to children. Adults would be scandalised and outraged if a police officer were to slap them. But, of course, it's different.

Isn't it a matter of degree? Certainly the severe abuse of a child brings about a public response of fury and condemnation. A key case in the history of child protection was that of Maria Colwell:

> The post-mortem carried out by Professor Cameron on 11 January [1973] showed that she was severely bruised all over the body and head and had sustained severe internal injuries to the stomach. There was a healing fracture of one rib. The bruising, which was described by Professor Cameron as the worst he had ever seen, was of variable age up to 10 to 14 days at most, which was the longest period that bruising might be expected to last but the majority dated from within 48 hours. The majority of the injuries he described as the result of extreme violence. (DHSS 1973: 59–60)

There is no moral dilemma here. The violent death of Maria Colwell at the hands of her stepfather led to the general establishment of Child Abuse Registers, and it is worth noting that this is typical of the history of child protection: major policy changes coming about as a result of a particularly dramatic case.

But legislation alone does not control violence (if indeed, it can be controlled). Writing in 1968 Radbill commented:

No parent now has the right to kill his child, and there is no distinction between infanticide and murder. The legal limits to chastisement of children, however, are not clearcut; such limitations have to be supplemented by public opinion. (p. 6)

Abusive parenting exists in, and is subject to modification by, the current ethos regarding the rights of adults to punish children physically. Garbarino (1977) suggests that society's sanctioning of the physical punishment of children is one of the necessary preconditions of abuse. The severe punishment of children in schools, with the cane and the strap, was general in the UK twenty years ago and was not abolished in state-funded schools until 1987 (Leach, 1993).

What is permissible in the wider society is the standard against which individual parents' treatment of their children is measured and judged and, to some extent, by which they judge themselves. This moral relativity at any one time, and over periods of history, has to be borne in mind when we attempt to assess the 'objective' scale of the problem.

CHILD ABUSE AND CHILD PROTECTION: THE HISTORICAL PERSPECTIVE

Pinchbeck and Hewitt (1973) in their historical review *Children in English Society* write that:

> until late in the nineteenth century, both Parliament and the national press were largely unconcerned with the way in which parents treated their children, regarding even the most barbarous cruelty as beyond comment and beyond public intervention since children were not then regarded as citizens in their own right. (p. 611)

The 'private' maltreatment of children was matched by public maltreatment, as part of the process of law:

> On one day alone, in February 1814, at the Old Bailey Sessions, five children were condemned to death; Fowler, aged twelve, and Wolfe, aged twelve, for burglary in a dwelling; Morris, aged eight, Solomons, aged nine, and Burrell, aged eleven, for burglary and stealing a pair of shoes. (Pinchbeck and Hewitt, 1973: 351–2)

Although society at that time was harsh for most people, the point is that little exception was made for children. The moves to restrict the employment of children, during the first half of the nineteenth century, made slow progress. For example the use of small boys to climb inside chimney flues, sentimentalised in Charles Kingsley's 1863 classic, *The Water Babies*, was not actually prohibited by Act of Parliament until 1874.

Public intervention into the private care of children was strongly resisted. It took a particularly flagrant scandal to turn public opinion and force legislative action.

The practice of abandoning babies (both dead and alive) was a major problem in all urban areas in the nineteenth century. The New York Foundling Hospital was established in 1869 and in the year 1873, 1,392 foundlings were left there (Radbill, 1968). But many infants were also found dead in the streets.

An identical situation obtained in London. In the year 1870 no fewer than 276 dead babies were found in London streets, most of them being under one week old (Pinchbeck and Hewitt, 1973). The problem was brought into focus by the practices of some 'baby farmers' who, having accepted payment for taking care of unwanted babies, murdered them and disposed of their bodies. The surrounding scandal led to the Infant Life Protection Act of 1872 which was further amended in 1887 following the execution of a notorious baby farmer, Mrs Dyer, the year before.

One of the better-known features of the history of child protection is that in both the UK and the US national societies for the prevention of cruelty to animals were established before societies for the prevention of cruelty to children. The full story is even more bizarre. In the US the first challenge to parental rights came about in New York in 1874 when the Society for the Prevention of Cruelty to Animals successfully prosecuted the adoptive parents of a girl, Mary Ellen, who had starved and brutally beaten her, on the basis that the child, as a member of the animal kingdom 'was entitled to at least the same justice as a common cur on the streets' (Fontana, 1971: 185).

In the UK the National Society for the Prevention of Cruelty to Children was established in 1889, having originated in Liverpool in 1882 when 'at a meeting organised by the society for the Prevention of Cruelty to Animals, an appeal for a Dogs' Home became extended into an appeal for the protection of children' (Pinchbeck and Hewitt, 1973: 621).

The 1889 Prevention of Cruelty to Children Act was the first piece of legislation targeted on the private treatment of children. It is sobering to reflect that this is little more than a hundred years ago. In the five years following, some six thousand people were prosecuted under the Acts. In 1908 a comprehensive Children's Act was established which sought to give children social rights independent of their parents. A revolution had occurred; but it was far from complete, and the vulnerability of children remained such that, even now, the questioning of parental treatment of their children is often seen as an infringement of human rights.

THE SCALE OF PHYSICAL ABUSE

The scale of adult violence towards children is unknown and, indeed, unknowable. Domestic violence is carried out in private and it is only when injury results or when children are articulate and confident enough to report abuse that it can be detected. Most violence does not result in conspicuous injury except in the case of the very young, and it is significant that the highest rates of reported and registered cases are in the under-5-years age range (Department of Health, 1994; Creighton, 1992). The lower reported rates in the older age ranges may simply be a function of their greater resilience: a 10-year-old will walk away from a blow that would kill a 1-year-old.

Serious injuries and fatalities are rarely unknown to professionals; but they may be misclassified. Moderate injuries are the most ambiguous; and violence not resulting in injury may attract no attention at all.

Not all abuse is detected, or recognised for what it is; not all abuse that *is* detected is reported to child protection agencies; not all of those cases reported are registered. Yet in the UK at least, our knowledge of the scale of abuse is based almost entirely on those cases which appear on Child Protection Registers. In other words we do not know the true scale of child abuse. *There is no UK research on the true prevalence and incidence of child abuse.*

Indeed, it is only since 1990 that the Department of Health started to collect (and publish in the form of Annual Reports) data on children registered from all Social Services Departments in England (but not Wales or Scotland). In the most recent report (Department of Health, 1994) and excluding the largely defunct 'at risk' category ('Grave Concern') 43 per cent of the children registered were classified as physically abused (p. 10) and of these children 36 per cent were under the age of 5 years. In relation to the population of children at large this gives a rate of only 6 per 10,000 of the under 18 population, which would be comfortingly low if it represented the true picture.

Is the situation improving? Child abuse cases receive much media publicity and Social Services Departments have for years been devoting a major part of their budgets to child protection. The nearest we can get to an answer is by referring to the NSPCC's longitudinal study, a unique record of research in the UK (Creighton, 1985; Creighton and Noyes, 1989; Creighton, 1992).

Until 1990 the NSPCC were responsible for maintaining Child Protection Registers in approximately 10 per cent of local authorities in England and Wales. These studies, although less geographically comprehensive than the Department of Health Reports, provide a much wider range of information, in particular in the analysis of the relationships between different kinds of data and other information available at a national level (employment levels; social class membership; family composition; and so on). In addition the studies are *longitudinal* in character, so giving us some evidence on which to judge changes.

As noted above, 0–4 year olds are particularly vulnerable to abuse and so rates in this age range probably give a sensitive indicator of trends. Figure 2.1 (from Creighton, 1992) shows the injury rates for this age-group from 1973–90. The figure shows an increase in injury rate between 1974 and 1975 followed by a marked decrease in 1976. It was at this time that Child Abuse Registers became generally established throughout the country (Jones *et al.*, 1979). This was a direct consequence of the death of Maria Colwell (described earlier) when the Inquiry Report (DHSS, 1973) revealed fundamental inadequacies in professional communication and supervision.

The Registers appear to have had an immediate effect, since there was now a central 'clearing house' to which suspicious professionals could refer. Previously, abusing parents had been known to 'hospital shop' – taking their injured child to different doctors and hospitals (Skinner and Castle, 1969). However, post-1978, as the economic recession began to deepen, injury rates show an erratic tendency to increase. There is certainly no evidence of a continuous improvement in the situation.

Over the 16-year period of the NSPCC study the average age of physically abused children (as registered) increased steadily – from 3 years

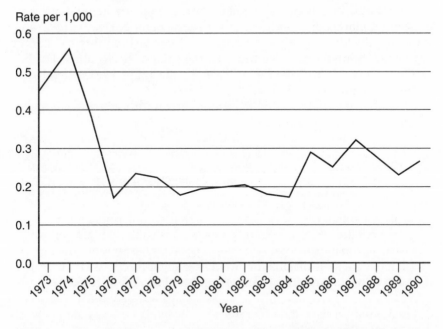

Figure 2.1 Fatal and serious injury for 0–4 year-olds in England and Wales: registered cases in NSPCC sample

Source: From Creighton, 1992, Figure 9

8 months in 1975 to 7 years 1 month in 1990. The reasons for this are not clear but a major factor was probably the initial emphasis on the un-recognised physical abuse of very young children – the so-called 'battered child syndrome'.

THE BATTERED CHILD SYNDROME

When a paper with this title was published in 1962 by Dr Henry Kempe and his associates at the University of Colorado School of Medicine, the public response was immediate.

Describing a condition of 'unrecognised trauma' in young children, the paper marked the beginning of a new era in child protection, fuelled by popular and professional feelings of guilt. For Kempe's paper was the culmination rather than the beginning of a process of research that had been steadily resisted. A similar problem is manifest today in reluctance to consider that some of the infant deaths recorded as Sudden Infant Death Syndrome (cot death) may be the result of abuse or neglect (Emery, 1985).

Yet the evidence had been there in the medical literature for almost twenty years. In 1946 Caffey, a radiologist, described cases of multiple fractures in the long bones of infants suffering from subdural hematoma (bleeding underneath the intracranial covering of the brain). He had been collecting such cases for a period of some twenty years. Silverman (1953) described a very similar case and observed that 'The roentgen [X-ray] diagnosis of traumatic lesions was strongly resisted by pediatricians and orthopedists interested in the child' (p. 417).

A paper by Woolley and Evans (1955) described twelve such cases and commented:

> An extremely important point to be noted is that when these infants were removed from their environments for periods varying from a week to several months no new lesions developed and those that were already present healed at the expected rate. (p. 54)

From this point on the level of professional (if not public) awareness increased rapidly, although Kempe's paper was still seven years away.

This incursion into the past is to make a point for the present. Not only do we not know the scale of abuse but we do not always recognise it for what it is when we see it. And in this respect professionals are as culpable as the public; if not more so because of their knowledge and privileged access.

WHO ARE THE ABUSED AND WHO ARE THE ABUSERS?

We have seen that younger children are more likely to be physically injured than older children. A general finding is that boys are more likely than girls to be physically abused – the reverse being the case in sexual abuse (Creighton, 1992; Department of Health, 1994).

Overwhelmingly, *physically* abused children are from the poorer and disadvantaged sections of society. And even within the norms for the manual social classes they are twice as likely to be living with only one of their natural parents (Creighton, 1992: 25). The parental situation of physically injured children is shown in Figure 2.2.

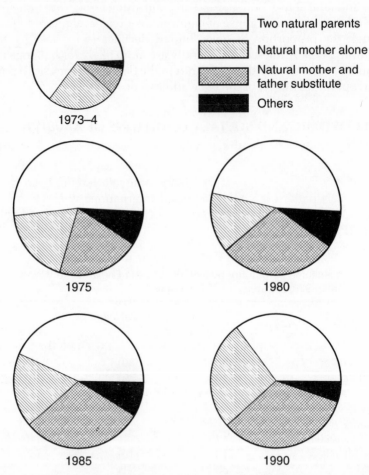

Figure 2.2 The parental situation of injured children in England and Wales 1975–90: NSPCC sample

Source: From Creighton, 1992, Figure 11

The same study shows that the perpetrator of the abuse is as likely to be the natural mother (30 per cent of cases) as the natural father (29 per cent) but this has to be qualified in a number of important respects:

- abused children are *twice* as likely to be living with their natural mother as their natural father, i.e. the 'risk' is not equivalent;
- even when the natural father is present the natural mother is still likely to bear the brunt of child care, i.e. their *exposure* to the stresses and strains of child-rearing is disproportionate.

The other large category of perpetrator (10 per cent) is that of father substitutes who are more likely than natural fathers to be involved in severe and fatal abuse. Both natural and substitute fathers are more often involved in the physical abuse of children over ten (Creighton, 1992: 33), although the proportion of boys injured declines (see Table 2.1 from Creighton, 1992). Adolescents generally are more likely to challenge their parents but quite simply there is a shift in the balance of (physical) power – in favour, particularly, of the male adolescent.

THE ECONOMIC AND SOCIAL CONDITIONS OF ABUSIVE FAMILIES

The overwhelming picture is that abusive families are those in which the father is in a manual occupation (or unemployed, having been so employed). This pattern is widely reported internationally and cannot be explained away by reporting bias, particularly in the case of severe injuries (Pelton, 1978).

Table 2.1 Suspected perpetrator by type of abuse in England and Wales, 1988–90 combined: NSPCC sample

Perpetrator		Physical injury	
	No.	%	% l.w.
Natural mother	831	(30)	(33)
Natural father	813	(29)	(61)
Both	93	(3)	(4)
Stepmother	24	(1)	(40)
Stepfather	220	(8)	(63)
Mother substitute	13		(10)
Father substitute	275	(10)	(59)
Sibling	32	(1)	
Other relative	42	(2)	
Other	111	(4)	
Total	2454	(88)	
No information	332	(12)	

Source: From Creighton, 1992, Table 17
Notes: l.w. = living with

In summary the parents of physically abused children are more likely to:

- be lone or in a 'reconstituted' partnership;
- be unemployed;
- be of low socioeconomic status;
- be of poor education;
- be teenage at the time of the *birth* of the abused child;
- have a criminal record, even with these other factors taken into account.

(Creighton, 1992)

It would be too easy for this to be taken as explaining abuse in terms of the personal characteristics of abusers – not that these should be disregarded. But the point is that all of the factors listed above are highly correlated with poverty and other forms of social disadvantage – in the family and in the area where they live. These factors can be seen as indices of or 'proxies' for poverty. Poverty is not a sufficient explanation of child abuse (most poor parents do not abuse their children) but it is likely to be a necessary one in most cases.

THE CAUSES OF CHILD ABUSE

In the 1960s and the early 1970s there was a great deal of research aimed at identifying the 'personality defects' of abusing (or potentially abusing) parents, e.g. Green *et al.* (1974). What is notable in this early literature is a reluctance to accept the evidence that severe child abuse and neglect is strongly related to socioeconomic status and outright poverty.

The main argument against this has been that the poor are more subject to public scrutiny than the professional and managerial classes. Discussing this 'public scrutiny' theory Pelton (1978) advances three counterarguments:

- First, while it is generally acknowledged that greater public awareness and new reporting laws have led to a significant increase in reporting over the past few years, the socioeconomic pattern of these reports has not changed appreciably.
- Second [it] cannot explain why child abuse and neglect are related to *degrees* of poverty, even *within* the same lower class that is acknowledged to be more open to public scrutiny.
- Third [it] cannot explain why, among the reported cases, the most severe injuries have occurred within the poorest families.

If the prevention of child abuse depends upon the elimination of poverty (however desirable that may be), then the prospects do not look very good. However, the picture is not that simple. Although poverty may be a usually-necessary precondition, it is not sufficient. Other factors have to operate: at the level of the individual parent, the family unit, the local neighbourhood, and the wider culture. This multi-layered perspective is conventionally referred to as *ecological*.

A first question to ask is: where is child abuse to be found? Cotterill (1988) mapped all households which had one or more children registered as abused or neglected (mostly cases of physical abuse) in an inner London borough between January 1982 and September 1985. He showed that there were clear concentrations of cases in particular areas:

> These 16 areas [of 7 or more cases] contained 73 per cent of the cases registered over the study period. The areas were of small size, none larger than half a mile across. Of the 16 areas, 12 were housing estates. (p. 466)

A key theoretical paper taking the ecological perspective is that of Garbarino (1977). There is not space here to replicate its arguments but it is recommended reading. In summary he argues that:

> Almost no-one is immune to the *role* of child abuse if the discrepancy between situational demands (e.g. difficulty of the child, emotional stress on the caregiver, etc) is great enough, although people vary in the degree to which they are 'prone' to act in an abusive manner. (p. 723)

Garbarino makes the important distinction between the *sufficient* and *necessary* conditions for child abuse to occur, observing that 'the absence of required necessary conditions effectively 'disarms' the sufficient conditions' (p. 725). He suggests that there are *two* necessary conditions and that both are best understood within an ecological framework:

- 'First, for child abuse to occur within family microsystems there must be cultural justification for the use of force against children' (p. 725).
- 'Of equal or greater importance on a day-to-day basis . . . is *isolation from potent support systems*' (p. 726).

He based his argument on his empirical research in New York State where he found that 'the degree to which mothers . . . are subjected to socioeconomic stress, *without adequate support systems*, accounts for a substantial proportion of the variance in rates of maltreatment' (p. 607).

'Support' takes many forms and has a number of consequences. In the UK Brown and Harris (1978) in an epidemiological study of depression in women (which they found to be more common in those with small children) also found that interpersonal supports (close relationships) were a major protection against depressive illness in the face of stressful life events.

Social support systems also regulate behaviour. Caplan (1974) suggests that they tell the individual 'what is expected of him and guide him in what to do. They watch what he does and they judge his performance' (p. 605). This reflects Garbarino's (1977) notion that 'child abuse "feeds" on privacy' (p. 727).

Garbarino and Sherman (1980) in later empirical work found that families 'who need the most tend to be clustered together in settings that must struggle to meet their needs' (p. 194) – a finding mirrored in Cotterill's research cited above. They conclude: 'we have the repeated finding that ecological niches can "make or break" risky families' (p. 196). In other words some families, some individuals, are *predisposed* to abuse, but whether they *do* depends on a number of other conditions.

Belsky (1980) draws attention to the *individual characteristics of children* as a predisposing factor in abuse. He points out that a repeated finding is that often just one child in a family is singled out for abuse, and the intuitively unlikely finding that a disproportionate number of maltreated children are born prematurely. Douglas (1989) writing about the problem of crying babies reports research that shows that the crying of premature infants is different from those born full-term, and is more likely to arouse negative reactions in adults. She comments: 'it could be that the more aversive a baby's cries are the less parents can tolerate it and start to feel increasingly stressed and upset' (p. 178). In short, there are no single, simple causes of abuse; a number of factors have to come together to take the caretaking adults above their threshold of tolerance.

THE EFFECTS OF ABUSE

Some forms of non-accidental injury have lasting effects (it is, for example, a significant cause of blindness in children) but young bodies heal very quickly. However, if there are usually no long-term physical effects what about psychological injury? Are these children emotionally and socially impaired?

A much-promoted notion, dating specifically from Kempe's 1962 paper, is that abused children become abusing parents (or that abusing parents have necessarily been abused themselves). There is more evidence for the latter than for the former: but they are not the same thing.

There is a lesson here in the need to scrutinise research methods and the inferences drawn from them. In this case the difference between the *retrospective* method and the *prospective* method. In the first of these you take a group of abusing parents and find out what percentage of them were abused as children; in the second method you follow up a group of adults, abused in childhood, before or at the point where they become parents themselves to see whether they abuse their children. Any association is maximised by the first method (because it excludes parents who were abused but didn't become abusers). Because the hypothesis of 'intergenerational transmission' is so highly promoted it is worth reviewing a prospective study to show the difference in the association depending on the method used.

Hunter and Kilstrom (1979) interviewed 282 parents of newborn babies and followed them up for one year, checking on registered cases of neglect and abuse. At the initial interview 49 parents reported a childhood history of abuse or neglect. At the follow-up, ten babies were reportedly maltreated: nine of them had parents with a history of abuse and neglect. This is a highly significant overlap, but the fact remains that 40 parents with a history of abuse and neglect were *not* identified as maltreaters.

Kaufman and Zigler (1987), comment on this study:

> If [it] had been conducted retrospectively with only the parents who were identified as maltreaters, the link between a history of abuse and subsequent child abuse would have appeared deceptively strong, since nine out of ten of the abusive parents reported a history of maltreatment (90 per cent). By employing a prospective research design, Hunter and Kilstrom were able to identify 40 parents who broke the cycle of abuse (82 per cent). (p. 188)

Aggregating a number of studies Kaufman and Zigler concluded that the best estimate of the 'intergenerational transmission' rate is 30 per cent ± 5 per cent. They conclude that we should 'cease asking "Do abused children become abusive parents?" and ask, instead, "Under what conditions is the transmission of abuse most likely to occur?"' (p. 191).

Translated into research terms, a beginning is to ask what the psychological effects are on children and to what extent they are persistent.

THE PSYCHOLOGICAL CHARACTERISTICS OF ABUSED CHILDREN

There is no doubt that abused children display more behavioural and emotional disorders than non-abused children, even when matched in other respects. There is equally no doubt that the disorders are non-specific, i.e. there is no particular personality profile or pattern of disorders which distinguishes abused children. Physical abuse is one of a number of possible causes for the same 'symptoms'.

However, there is widespread agreement of consistently high levels of aggression in abused children. Early clinical studies reported this, e.g. Elmer and Gregg (1967), as have later controlled studies. Reidy (1977) looked at the aggressive characteristics of 20 physically abused, 16 non-abused but neglected and 22 non-maltreated children with average ages of 6½–7 years. Abused children displayed more fantasy aggression in projective tests and very much more overt aggression in play situations. In the latter context both neglected and non-abused children displayed hardly any aggressive behaviour. Herrenkohl and Herrenkohl (1981) in a larger study found essentially similar results but noted that the maltreated children's aggression was chiefly in response to 'difficult' tasks or 'interference' from their peers.

But we must avoid any simple equation, e.g. abused child = aggression. The danger lies in over-generalisation from a consistent trend. In the same way that parents with a history of abuse in childhood are more likely to maltreat their children, so are maltreated children more likely to be aggressive. But most individuals avoid this 'causal' pattern; and even where it is true there is more to the outcome than heightened aggressive or abusive tendencies. The consequences of abuse (or any other adverse experience) are *mediated*: filtered and changed by the individual's response and by the kinds of help and understanding they are given.

Recent research, e.g. Cowen and Work (1988) emphasises the concept of *resilience*: the process (however it operates) by which children overcome adverse experiences. 'Risk' factors have to be counterbalanced by 'protective' factors. Rutter (1987) comments: 'protection . . . resides, not in the evasion of risk, but in successful engagement with it' (p. 318) and adds 'interaction effects are crucial for protective processes' (p. 319).

Rutter reviews the operation of these processes in relation to the differential effects of marital discord on boys as opposed to girls. Marital discord is frequently noted as a high frequency factor in child abuse cases (e.g. Creighton, 1992: 20). Rutter suggests a number of reasons such as greater male vulnerability, parents being more likely to quarrel in front of boys, boys more likely to react aggressively and be treated more punitively. In other words there are many components to the concepts of risk and invulnerability.

The main damage in psychological terms may lie in the extent to which two fundamental needs of all human beings are not satisfied:

- the need to be valued in a secure and harmonious love relationship (a fundamental for later successful relationships and something which abused and neglected children are likely to lack in most but not all cases);
- the need to accomplish successfully tasks which the individual sees as important (something which abused children are impaired in achieving, as noted earlier).

The implications of such impairments are general, affecting the ability to make relationships, to learn, and to cope with work and task demands; and so are fundamentally disabling.

REFERENCES

Belsky, J. (1980) 'Child maltreatment: an ecological integration', *American Psychologist* 35: 320–35.

Brown, G.W. and Harris, T. (1978) *Social Origins of Depression: A Study of Psychiatric Disorder in Women*, London: Tavistock.

Caffey, J. (1946) 'Multiple fractures in long bones of infants suffering from chronic subdural hematoma', *American Journal of Roentgenology* 56: 163–73.

Caplan, G. (1974) *Support Systems and Community Mental Health*, New York: Behavioural Publications.

Cotterill, A.M. (1988) 'The geographic distribution of child abuse in an inner city borough', *Child Abuse and Neglect* 12: 461–7.

Cowen, E.L. and Work, W.C. (1988) 'Resilient children, psychological wellness and primary prevention', *American Journal of Community Psychology* 16: 591–607.

Creighton, S.J. (1985) 'An epidemiological study of abused children and their families in the United Kingdom between 1977 and 1982', *Child Abuse and Neglect* 9: 441–8.

—— (1992) *Child Abuse Trends in England and Wales 1988–1990*, London: NSPCC.

Creighton, S.J. and Noyes, P. (1989) *Child Abuse Trends in England and Wales 1983–1987*, London: NSPCC.

Department of Health (1994) *Children and Young People on Child Protection Registers Year Ending 31 March 1993 England*, London: Government Statistical Service.

DHSS (1973) *Report of the Committee of Inquiry into the Care and Supervision Provided in Relation to Maria Colwell*, London: HMSO.

Douglas, J. (1989) *Behaviour Problems in Young Children*, London: Routledge.

Elmer, E. and Gregg, G. (1967) 'Developmental characteristics of abused children', *Pediatrics* 40: 596–602.

Emery, J.L. (1985) 'Infanticide, filicide and cot death', *Archives of Disease in Childhood* 60: 505–7.

Fontana, V.J. (1971) *The Maltreated Child* (2nd edition), Springfield, Ill.: Charles C. Thomas.

Garbarino, J. (1977) 'The human ecology of child maltreatment: a conceptual model for research', *Journal of Marriage and the Family* 39: 721–7.

Garbarino, J. and Sherman, D. (1980) 'High-risk neighbourhoods and high-risk families: the human ecology of child maltreatment', *Child Development* 51: 188–98.

Green, A.H., Gaines, R.W. and Sandgrund, A. (1974) 'Child abuse: pathological syndrome of family interaction', *American Journal of Psychiatry* 131: 882–6.

Herrenkohl, R.C. and Herrenkohl, E.C. (1981) 'Some antecedents and developmental consequences of child maltreatment', *New Directions for Child Development* 11: 57–76.

Hunter, R. and Kilstrom, N. (1979) 'Breaking the cycle of abusive families', *American Journal of Psychiatry* 136: 1320–2.

Jones, D.N., Hill, K.P. and Thorpe, R. (1979) 'Central child abuse registers: the British experience', *Child Abuse and Neglect* 3: 157–66.

Kaufman, J. and Zigler, E. (1987) 'Do abused children become abusive parents?', *American Journal of Orthopsychiatry* 57, 2: 186–92.

Kempe, C.H., Silverman, F.N., Stelle, B.F., Droegemuller, W. and Silver, H.K. (1962) 'The battered-child syndrome', *Journal of the American Medical Association* 181, 1: 17–24.

Leach, P. (1993) 'Should parents hit their children?', *The Psychologist* 6, 5: 216–20.

Pelton, L.H. (1978) 'Child abuse and neglect: the myth of classlessness', *American Journal of Orthopsychiatry* 48: 608–17.

Pinchbeck, I. and Hewitt, M. (1973) *Children in English Society* (Volume II), London: Routledge and Kegan Paul.

Radbill, S.X. (1968) 'A history of child abuse and infanticide', in R.E. Helfer and C.H. Kempe (eds), *The Battered Child*, Chicago: University of Chicago Press.

Reidy, T. (1977) 'The aggressive characteristics of abused and neglected children', *Journal of Clinical Psychology* 33: 1140–5.

Rutter, M. (1987) 'Psychosocial resilience and protective mechanisms', *American Journal of Orthopsychiatry* 57, 3: 316–31.

Silverman, F. (1953) 'Roentgen manifestations of unrecognized skeletal trauma in infants', *American Journal of Roentgenology* 69: 413–26.

Skinner, A.E. and Castle, R.L. (1969) *78 Battered Children: A Retrospective Study,* London: NSPCC.

Woolley, P.V. and Evans, W.A. (1955) 'Significance of skeletal lesions in infants resembling those of traumatic origin', *Journal of the American Medical Association* 158: 539–43.

Chapter 3

The prevention of child abuse

Bill Gillham

The previous chapter began with an account of the death of Maria Colwell in the early 1970s. At the end of that decade the UK Department of Health published *A Study of Inquiry Reports 1973–81* dealing with eighteen investigations (Department of Health, 1982). These were all headline cases of fatal child abuse. Another decade later *A Study of Inquiry Reports 1980–89* (Department of Health, 1991) was published covering nineteen such investigations.

This later publication reviews progress in preventing serious abuse: the introduction comments:

> What was remarkable in the first decade of inquiries was the coherence of the findings. In the 1980s a more complicated picture emerges. The messages from the last decade of reports may seem depressing but it is understandable where difficult decisions concerning human relationships are being made by professional staff from a number of agencies that tragedies will from time to time occur. (p. iii)

Implied here is that the task of prevention, at least in the sense of identifying specific cases, is impossible. The report quotes from an investigation into the death of one child as follows:

> It was said to us before we started hearing evidence that if we could suggest ways in which families like this, who in no way stand out from hundreds of others with whom the agencies deal, could somehow be identified before the tragedy occurs it would be an enormous help. It will be clear from the pages that follow that although we suggest ways in which practice might be improved, we have been unable to suggest any infallible method of spotting potential child killers. (p. 63)

An American researcher, Alfaro, reviewing nine US studies of child abuse fatalities puts the matter even more succinctly:

> The demand that fatalities and serious harm be prevented assumes that the means of prediction and prevention exist. Hindsight reviews

of fatality cases frequently create the impression that the precursors to death were clearly visible and that a timely and effective intervention might have saved a life. (Alfaro, 1991: 219)

If we can't identify cases with the most serious outcomes, what chance have we of detecting potential cases of 'mild' abuse? We know what the risk factors are; but the overwhelming majority of parents 'at risk' of abusing treat their children perfectly well.

But even if we *knew* that abuse was going to happen it does not follow that we could mount an effective intervention (unless the 'risk' factors could be modified). Knowing that something is going to happen doesn't mean that you can stop it. Many teachers and others can see adolescents sliding into delinquency. But what can they (or anyone else) do about it?

These are intended to be tough rather than negative or pessimistic questions. We have to ask *how* we can help and *what* we can change. Consider this by no means exhaustive list of risk factors for child abuse:

• parental history of abuse
• parental criminal record
• marital discord
• low income
• manual occupation or unemployed
• 'reconstituted' partnership
• 'difficult' child
• living in a socially disadvantaged area
• social isolation
• maternal depression

How many of these factors can we do anything about? The issue needs to be examined in more detail before any programme of action can be outlined.

THINKING ABOUT PREVENTION

The practical problems of tackling child abuse can seem overwhelming. A first step is to consider what is meant by 'prevention'; and then to focus on what might be achievable.

A much over-used public health model of prevention is as follows:

• *primary* (before it happens)
• *secondary* (early treatment)
• *tertiary* (minimising effects)

This kind of model works best in dealing with health problems where probable *causes*, numbers of *cases*, and the effectiveness of *treatments* can be specified (see discussion in Giovannoni, 1982: 23–4).

In relation to child abuse, primary prevention hardly exists (even if it were practicable). Child-protection services are hard-pressed to deal with those cases that are referred to them after the event. Social workers work hard, and often imaginatively, to attempt to reduce the risk of further abuse, but are limited in the scale of what they can do by their case-load. However, it is probable that child protection services, by their very existence, have some regulating effect.

One point to keep in mind when considering 'primary risk' is that *correlates* are not necessarily *causes*. Lone parents, young mothers, those in manual occupations, and the unemployed are over-represented on child protection registers. What they have in common is poverty, and a consistent research finding is that where these other factors are controlled for, it is being poor that surfaces as the fundamental social cause.

Because child abuse is embedded in large-scale social problems endemic in our society, child abuse is endemic. That does not render us powerless, but it is essential to be realistic. To be otherwise is to deny the nature of the problem. The consequences of poverty and unemployment are many: child abuse is only part of the pattern (Steinberg *et al.*, 1981).

Gordon (1983) suggests that we should abandon the 'health' model of prevention in relation to social problems and think in terms of:

- *universal* measures (that benefit everybody)
- *selective* measures (for high-risk groups)
- *indicated* measures (for identified families or individuals)

Large-scale problems require universal measures through large-scale political action. Professions such as psychology and education and social work cannot operate at this level. It does not mean, however, that they should not seek to inform and influence policy and public awareness.

Poor social conditions for parents and children are one side of the equation. On the other is the problem of parents who have children too early in their lives: as noted in the previous chapter, abused children are much more likely to have been born when their mother was under the age of twenty. Such parents are not so much inadequate personally, as inadequate in their resources for the role in which they find themselves. The 1986 survey *Teenage Mothers and Their Partners* commissioned by the DHSS is particularly illuminating in this respect (Simms and Smith, 1986).

Teenage pregnancies have declined proportionately in all Western societies over the past twenty years or so (Jones, *et al.*, 1986) but they are most likely to occur in the most socially disadvantaged groups (Smith, 1993). And working class young mothers are less likely than middle-class ones to seek (or be encouraged to seek) abortion (Smith, 1993). The UK Government is aware of the problem in that it has set targets for reducing teenage pregnancies (Secretary of State for Health, 1992). But in practice, imaginative attempts to provide more effective contraception advice for teenagers often fall foul of political sensitivity to what is implied (Ashton, 1989).

There is little doubt that a reduction in teenage pregnancies would have an impact on child abuse rates; and also on related problems of mental health in young women – particularly *depression* (Paykel, 1991), which is extremely common and itself has serious effects on children (i.e. the 'psychologically unavailable' mother) (Farber and Egeland, 1987: 266).

Educationists might tend to see a 'universal' approach as one that focused on education and child care programmes for teenagers. These are 'face valid' like most social education programmes but there is absolutely no evidence that they make young people more sexually responsible or better at parenting. Social education programmes are flawed in that they assume a more rational basis for behaviour than is actually the case (Ingham, 1994). This lack of effectiveness of educational programmes in relation to actual *behaviour* has been demonstrated elsewhere – for example in relation to drug abuse by adolescents (Davies and Coggans, 1991: 61) and child pedestrian safety (Thomson, 1991: 71). Children and young people learn more about the risks and what they *should* do; but there appears to be little direct effect on actual behaviour. Educationists' faith in these 'knowledge enhancement' approaches represents a fundamental misconception of the determinants of human behaviour – at least in the young.

'Universal' social improvements that affect everybody are particularly important for parents with the potential for physical abuse. One can see that process at work when national economies improve (or decline). Such universal changes mean that one does not have to deal with the problems involved in 'selective' intervention which involve identifying high-risk populations of parents *before* abuse occurs and providing forms of support which are predicted to reduce the likelihood. There are serious difficulties with this approach. In the first place it is stigmatic. However presented, parents are essentially being 'accused' of being abusers, withall potentially. One has to be on the receiving end of such suspicion to discover how offensive it is (see Howitt, 1992). Secondly, assuming a population base rate of abuse at around 1 per cent, even with very good predictors (which we don't have), two things happen:

- *some* parents who will abuse are not identified (false negatives)
- *very many* parents who will not abuse are identified (false positives)

A compromise solution is to adopt a 'selective universal' approach to identifying groups of parents, particularly mothers, who are significantly at risk (e.g. young, single, poor, with children under two) but who also demonstrably need support on simple humane grounds.

There are a number of reasons why such a selective emphasis should focus on parents with very young children. We know that the most severe forms of child abuse occur in the under-two age-range (the 'battered child' syndrome). There is also good reason to believe that some abuse of babies and young children is concealed under the 'diagnosis' of sudden infant death syndrome (SIDS) or 'near-miss' SIDS or other medical conditions, real or alleged, such as 'Munchausen syndrome by proxy' (Emery, 1985; Meadow, 1984). Thirdly, and relatedly, it is the mothers of such children (especially undersupported working-class mothers) who are particularly vulnerable to depression (Brown and Harris, 1978). We shall discuss this 'mental health' problem more fully later.

Garbarino and Crouter (1978) contended that 'child maltreatment is an indicator of the overall quality of life for children and families' (p. 607). If that is true then improving the quality of life for this vulnerable group is high priority and *not just because of the child abuse risk.*

The relationship between mothers and their babies is an intensely powerful one and capable of being very disturbing. It is not simply a matter of the equity or inequity of partners in child care. The fact that mothers can kill or injure their defenceless babies is the strongest evidence for the emotional character of the relationship. A major theoretical strand in the literature on child abuse concerns the role of *attachment*: the mutual pleasure and security that the mother and child derive from each other. This is not just the mother being 'attached' to the child: it is a two-way process and not firmly in place until the middle of the first year of life when the child shows clear evidence of recognition and preference for the mother. In attachment theory the absence or disruption of this bond means that the inhibitors that usually prevent maltreatment are not in place. This could partly explain the peculiar vulnerability of young babies to abuse.

Attachment is at the root of what has been called the 'irrational commitment' of parents: the ability to tolerate difficult behaviour and to go to unreasonable lengths to cope with the child's demands. The *quality* of attachment affects not only the particular child–adult relationship but the resilience of the family. Crittenden and Ainsworth (1989) suggest that insecure attachment relationships, apart from being mutually unsatisfactory, render all members of a family more vulnerable to external stresses such as poverty and unemployment, and so affect the ability to maintain stable relationships.

The probable long-term effects as well as the short-term misery make social support for the parents of young children a high priority. Belsky (1980) suggests that social support works in three main ways:

- by providing *emotional* support
- by providing *practical* help
- by reinforcing *social expectations* of 'good' parenting

This is most economically and satisfactorily provided by the immediate family and local community but a consistent finding is that *professional* support has positive effects on vulnerable groups of parents.

SELECTIVE SUPPORT FOR MOTHERS AND YOUNG CHILDREN

A strong finding is that home-visiting by nurses of mothers and babies (called 'health visitors' in the UK) reduces the risk of abuse, particularly serious abuse. Health visitors probably provide all the kinds of social support listed above, but the regulatory function of routine inspection of babies by professionals should not be underrated. Social control in an acceptable, non-stigmatic guise is a form of support. Babies and very young children can have 'low visibility' – the privacy that makes abuse both more likely and more easily concealed. We shall return to this point later in considering the regulatory functions of schools and nurseries.

Gray *et al.* (1977) were the first to carry out a well-designed controlled intervention study. They identified 100 high-risk mothers *before* the birth of their babies and randomly assigned them to either an intervention or control group. Intervention started at birth and involved greater contact with health workers generally and weekly nurse home-visiting. At follow-up when the children were aged 17–35 months they found no serious maltreatment in the intervention group whereas five children (10 per cent) of the control group had been hospitalised because of injuries. Another study by Crockenburg (1985) is particularly interesting because he compared groups of teenage mothers in the US and the UK, the latter group getting regular health visitor support. Most noticeably the young mothers in the English group were very much more positive and responsive in their behaviour towards their babies, a fundamental of good relationships.

In the UK such home support has been taken for granted. The importance of maintaining this service as a factor in preventing abuse and neglect is particularly apparent from US research where such a service has not been general practice. The most sophisticated study is that of Olds and his associates (Olds *et al.*, 1986). Because such well-designed studies are rare, and because the lessons are important we shall consider this in a little detail.

Some 400 women were enrolled in the study, *before* their first baby was born if they had any one of three 'risk' characteristics:

- age under nineteen
- single parent
- low socio-economic status

It was therefore a *prospective* study. The research team assumed that those at greatest risk would have all three characteristics: 23 per cent were in this category. The mothers were assigned to one of four treatment conditions:

1 a control group that participated only in data collection before and after
2 a group that only received transport for medical appointments
3 a group that received extensive *pre*natal nurse home-visiting and transport for subsequent medical appointments
4 a group that received extensive nurse home-visiting *post*natally as well as the services provided to group 3

The authors found that for the mothers at greatest risk (teenage *and* single *and* poor) the effect of nurse-visiting was greatest: 19 per cent of the mothers in the control group had abused or neglected their children in the first two years of life as against 4 per cent in the nurse-visited group. The authors observe:

> Although the treatment contrasts for the groups at lower risk did not reach statistical significance, virtually all of the contrasts were in the expected direction. Moreover, in the comparison condition the incidence of abuse and neglect increased as the number of risk factors accumulated, but in the nurse-visited condition, the incidence of abuse and neglect remained relatively low, even in those groups at higher risk. Also, the incidence of maltreatment in treatment 3 (nurse-visited: pregnancy) in general, was between the infancy nurse-visited and comparison conditions. (p. 71)

They go on to make the following interesting comment:

> The nurse-visited women reported less crying and fussiness on the part of their babies. Because reports of temperament and behavioral problems may be just as much a reflection of the mother's characteristics as the child's, we interpret reports of excessive crying and irritability as a problem in the parent–child relationship. (p. 76)

This last point reflects another aspect of the 'quality of relationship' effect of nurse home-visiting reported by Crockenburg and cited above.

More recently Olds and his associates carried out a follow-up study for the two-year period following the nurse home visiting which took place during the first two years of the children's lives (Olds *et al.*, 1994). They found no differences between the nurse-visited and comparison families for formally recorded abuse and neglect. But they did find that the 'visited' group had 40 per cent fewer injuries and 'ingestions' (accidental poisoning, etc.), made 35 per cent fewer visits to the hospital emergency department, and that 45 per cent fewer behavioural and parental coping problems were noted in the physician record. Interestingly the nurse-visited parents were observed to punish their children more often, but this appeared to be associated with the maintenance of standards, i.e. its 'functional' meaning was not abusive.

INDICATED PREVENTION: THE MENTAL HEALTH EFFECTS OF SOCIAL STRESS

Coping with children is a very demanding job. It requires physical and mental health in the parent; otherwise the insistent demands of children can become intolerable. Even something as mild as a headache, or the kind of mood swing that occurs as a matter of course, can make a parent more punitive than they would want to be. In the child-rearing age-range, and particularly for women, the major health problems are mental, not physical. And the major mental health problem for women is depression: 'the most persistent disorder in psychiatry' (Paykel, 1991: 22).

This chapter has stressed the need for social and societal intervention and prevention; but the presence or absence of these external factors has to be translated into psychological effects on the individual parent for abuse to occur. Parents are not equal even in similar circumstances. There are differences in character structure here (unfashionable levels of explanation: see Seagull, 1987). Some parents can absorb more stress or react to it more productively.

There are also important sex differences. Why do women (particularly women between twenty and forty and with children) report more depression than men in the same age and situation? Differences in role are part of the explanation. But it is also likely that men 'may differ in the way distress gets acknowledged and directed: into depression in females, in other ways and disorders in males' (Paykel, 1991: 22). For example, antisocial disorders are much more common in males and this is apparent from childhood (Rutter *et al.*, 1970). In the age-range where depression is more common in women, suicide (self-violence) is proportionally much more common in men (Hawton, 1987).

The relationship between the male's greater tendency to react violently to psychological distress and the physical abuse of children is an obvious one. The relationship between female depression and child abuse is less straightforward. It can operate in three ways:

- by making the mother 'psychologically unavailable' (see p. 30 above)
- by making her more intolerant of the demands of the child
- by making her less protective of the child (e.g. from a violent partner)

Studies of the social effects on mental health have focused almost exclusively on women (a fact to be noted); and a consistent finding is that it is having children that predisposes women to depression and related disorders. Gater *et al.* (1989) analysing the causes of higher psychiatric first admission rates for women, and looking at unmarried and married women with and without children found that having children accounted for the higher rates. However, emotional problems such as depression can arouse a helpful response in others in a way that aggressive behaviour does not; women are also more disposed to acknowledge their difficulties and seek help (Kessler *et al.*, 1981). The need for us to respond to problems that are acknowledged is clear. Less clear (and less attractive) is the need to help men with anger control and their violent expression of it. Public and official attitudes to men who physically harm children are severe in the extreme. Seeing violence as a clinical rather than just as a criminal problem is a significant shift in understanding. Howells and Hollin's (1989) book *Clinical Approaches to Violence* marks a constructive approach to this social problem. Identifying a substantial mental health problem does not necessarily mean a psychiatric response, or conventional notions of 'psychiatric' treatment. It does mean that we should understand some abusive behaviours for what they are.

PREVENTION: THE FACTOR OF 'VISIBILITY'

The high abuse rates of children under three are likely to be due to the specially stressful character of parenting at this stage and because young parents are less well-equipped to cope. But it is also the stage when children are least 'visible'. One function of regular professional visiting is to increase 'visibility'.

Once children reach nursery age (three plus) and as nursery provision increases (and it is often differentially allocated to socially disadvantaged children in the state sector in the UK) they become subject to daily scrutiny by teachers and nurses. The detection of suspicious bruising and other injuries is part of the regular training of such professionals and there are statutory procedures for notification. This vigilance, and parental knowledge of it, may act as a form of preventive social control. Nurseries and schools also provide parents with relief from the continuous care of children.

In the UK all children attend school from the age of five. When universal and compulsory education was established in Britain in 1870, one of the results was a clearer and heightened awareness of the physical and psychological condition of children. Social action followed, particularly the development of school health services and regular medical inspections (Pinchbeck and Hewitt, 1973). We now take the regulatory effects of this for granted but there can be no doubt that it is a very powerful means of protecting children. And the role of teachers is central: no other professional group regularly sees (and knows) *all* children. Preschool education is not yet universal but the benefits of this provision in terms of child protection should rank as high amongst the reasons for providing it.

INDICATED PREVENTION: VISIBLE INJURY

Writing as a paediatric consultant Speight (1993) observes:

Non-accidental injury is one of the most important diagnoses in clinical paediatrics as it can so vitally influence a child's future life. At worst it is a matter of life and death for the child and short of death there may still be possible brain damage or handicap. Though high risk cases are currently in a minority, the diagnosis remains crucially important in every case. This is because non-accidental injury is often a marker for emotional abuse and deprivation that can cause progressive and possibly permanent damage to a child's developing personality. This principle is especially relevant in children of school age. In such children the risk of death may be extremely small, yet non-accidental injury in older children is almost inevitably associated with a longstanding disturbance of the parent–child relationship. For this reason non-accidental injury should never be dismissed as 'over-chastisement'. (p. 5)

The key distinction is whether a perceived injury is 'accidental' or not. Exceptional injuries such as burns, scalds, fractures and lacerations are most likely to arouse suspicion. But the most usual visible evidence of abuse is bruising; and aren't bruises commonplace in children who play actively? Yes, they are but in two respects bruises are suspicious: if there are a number of them; and/or if their *location* on the body is unusual.

Bruises soon fade, usually in less than a week. Bruises also change colour very quickly so that some idea of how much bruising is going on can be judged by the *number* and *colour* of the bruises. For superficial bruising a rough guide is:

- less than 24 hours: red/purple
- 12–48 hours: purplish-blue
- 48–72 hours: brown
- more than 72 hours: yellow

(Speight, 1993)

Bruises on the shins are normal in all children but bruises to the head and neck; chest and abdomen; buttocks, arms and upper legs warrant more suspicion particularly if there are more than three bruises in one of these three areas (Sibert, 1994).

Injury in itself raises a question-mark: the kinds of injury and the number of them raise the level of suspicion. Other signs are:

- a recurrent pattern of injury though none in themselves is remarkable
- failure (or delay) on the part of parents to seek medical help
- vague or implausible or contradictory accounts of how the injuries occurred
- lack of appropriate concern
- aggressive or defensive behaviour (although innocent parents can behave in this way because they feel guilty)

Paediatric specialists can make distinctions beyond the competence of the layperson. But because injuries may be transient, the informed observations of those who first detect them – usually teachers or school nurses – can greatly assist the medical diagnosis and support the basis for subsequent social work action.

INDICATED PREVENTION: PROBLEM FAMILIES IN PROBLEM AREAS

There is good reason to believe (Oliver, 1983) that much abuse is concentrated in a number of problem families in well-defined areas, usually housing estates (Cotterill, 1988). Because the main drift of this chapter has been to emphasise the role of poverty and lack of social support as factors in child abuse, this does not mean that the individual characteristics of parents are not important. Most poor and poorly supported parents do not abuse their children and often provide for them remarkably well.

But using Gordon's classification, cited earlier, there are families (and areas) where professional input is *indicated*. Research being carried out by the author (Gillham and Toland, 1996, in preparation) which involves preparing geographical case-maps of registered cases of abuse and neglect in Glasgow, clearly shows concentrations of cases which persist from year to year: that is, the specific cases change to a large extent but they occur in approximately the same areas. Social workers (and teachers) do come to know these families well and work with them long-term to 'manage' their problems: this is the 'chronic' end of the continuum. But the larger-scale problem underlines the need for large-scale social improvements and high-quality universal prevention stemming from better support for all parents, and especially the parents of young children.

Once established, abusive patterns of interaction can be self-maintaining. Yet abusive parenting exists in, and is subject to modification by, the current ethos regarding the rights of adults to punish children physically. Children need to be controlled but there is no evidence that physical punishment works (Leach, 1993). As long as such punishment is considered justifiable then much physical abuse could be interpreted as legitimate. And if hitting children is a 'permitted' activity, it is easy for parents to go 'too far' in certain circumstances and so put themselves in the role of 'abuser'.

REFERENCES

Alfaro, J.D. (1991) 'What can we learn from child abuse fatalities? A synthesis of nine studies', in: D.J. Besharov (ed) *Protecting Children from Abuse and Neglect*, Springfield, Ill.: Charles C. Thomas.

Ashton, J. (1989) 'True story: the Liverpool project to reduce teenage pregnancy', *The British Journal of Family Planning* 15: 46–51.

Belsky, J. (1980) 'Child Maltreatment: An ecological integration', *American Psychologist* 35: 320–35.

—— (1984) 'The determinants of parenting: a processes model', *Child Development* 55: 83–96.

Brown, G.W. and Harris, T. (1978) *Social Origins of Depression: A Study of Psychiatric Disorder in Women*, London: Tavistock.

Cotterill, A.M. (1988) 'The geographic distribution of child abuse in an inner city borough', *Child Abuse and Neglect* 12: 461–7.

Crittenden, P.M. and Ainsworth, M.D.S. (1989) 'Child maltreatment and attachment theory', in D. Cicchetti and V. Carlson (eds), *Child Maltreatment*, New York: Cambridge University Press.

Crockenburg, S. (1985) 'Professional support and care of infants by adolescent mothers in England and the United States', *Journal of Pediatric Psychology* 10: 413–28.

Davies, J.B. and Coggans, N. (1991) *Adolescent Drug Abuse*, London: Cassell.

Department of Health (1982) *Child Abuse: A Study of Inquiry Reports 1973–1981*, London: HMSO.

Department of Health (1991) *Child Abuse: A Study of Inquiry Reports 1980–1989*, London: HMSO.

Emery, J.L. (1985) 'Infanticide, filicide and cot death', *Archives of Disease in Childhood* 60: 505–7.

Farber, E.A. and Egeland, B. (1987) 'Invulnerability among abused and neglected children', in E.J. Anthony and B.J. Cohler (eds), *The Invulnerable Child*, New York: Guilford Press.

Garbarino, J. and Crouter, A. (1978) 'Defining the community context for parent–child relations: the correlates of child maltreatment', *Child Development* 49: 604–16.

Gater, R.A., Dean, C. and Morris, J. (1989) 'The contribution of childbearing to the sex difference in first admission rates for affective psychosis', *Psychological Medicine* 19: 719–24.

Gillham, B. and Toland, A. (1996) 'Geographical density of registered cases of child physical abuse, sexual abuse and neglect in an urban area', (in preparation).

Giovannoni, J.M. (1982) 'Prevention of child abuse and neglect: research and policy issues', *Social Work Research and Abstracts* 18: 23–31.

Gordon, R.S. (1983) 'An operational classification of disease prevention', *Public Health Reports* 98: 107–9.

Gray, J.D., Cutler, C.A., Dean, J.G. and Kempe, C.H. (1977) 'Prediction and prevention of child abuse and neglect', *Child Abuse and Neglect* 1: 45–58.

Hawton, K. (1987) 'Assessment of suicide risk', *British Journal of Psychiatry* 150: 145–53.

Howells, K. and Hollin, C.R. (eds) (1989) *Clinical Approaches to Violence*, Chichester: John Wiley.

Howitt, D. (1992) *Child Abuse Errors*, London: Harvester Wheatsheaf.

Ingham, R. (1994) 'Some speculations on the concept of rationality', *Advances in Medical Sociology* 4: 89–111.

Jones, E.F. *et al.* (1986) *Teenage Pregnancy in Developed Countries*, New York: Yale University Press.

Kessler, R.C., Brown, R.L. and Broman, C.L. (1981) 'Sex differences in psychiatric help-seeking: evidence from four large-scale surveys', *Journal of Health and Social Behavior* 22: 49–64.

Leach, P. (1993) 'Should parents hit their children?', *The Psychologist* 6, 5: 216–20.

Meadow, R. (1984) 'Fictitious epilepsy', *The Lancet* 2: 25–8.

Olds, D.L., Henderson, C.R., Chamberlin, R. and Tatelbaum, R. (1986) 'Preventing child abuse and neglect: a randomized trial of nurse home visitation', *Pediatrics* 78, 1: 65–78.

Olds, D.L., Henderson, C.R. and Kitzman, H. (1994) 'Does prenatal and infancy nurse home visitation have enduring effects on qualities of parental caregiving and child health at 25 to 50 months of life?', *Pediatrics* 93, 1: 89–98

Oliver, J.E. (1983) 'Dead children from problem families in N.E. Wiltshire', *British Medical Journal* 286: 115–17.

Paykel, E.S. (1991) 'Depression in women', *British Journal of Psychiatry* 158, (suppl. 10): 22–9.

Pinchbeck, I. and Hewitt, M. (1973) *Children in English Society (Volume II)*, London: Routledge and Kegan Paul.

Rutter, M., Tizard, J. and Whitmore, K. (1970) *Education, Health and Behaviour*, London: Longman.

Seagull, E.A.W. (1987) 'Social support and child maltreatment: a review of the evidence', *Child Abuse and Neglect* 11: 41–52.

Secretary of State for Health (1992) *The Health of the Nation: A Strategy for Health in England*, London: HMSO.

Sibert, J. R. (1994) 'Mathematical models in diagnosing child abuse', Paper presented to the British Paediatric Association.

Simms, M. and Smith, C. (1986) *Teenage Mothers and Their Partners: A Survey in England and Wales* (Research Report No. 15) London: HMSO (for DHSS).

Smith, T. (1993) 'Influence of socioeconomic factors on attaining targets for reducing teenage pregnancies', *British Medical Journal* 306: 1232–5.

Speight, N. (1993) 'Non-accidental injury', in R. Meadow (ed.), *ABC of Child Abuse* (2nd edition), London: BMJ Publishing Group.

Steinberg, L.D., Catalano, R. and Dooley, D. (1981) 'Economic antecedents of child abuse and neglect', *Child Development* 52: 975–85.

Thomson, J. (1991) *Child Pedestrian Accidents*, London: Cassell.

Chapter 4

Child accidents at home, school and play

Helen Roberts

All small children have accidents, and children have accidents in the places where they spend the majority of their time. This means that they have accidents mainly in the home before the age of 5, and as they get older and spend more time outside the home, they increasingly have accidents in the wider environment. They have accidents in the spaces where they play, they have accidents at school and they have accidents on the roads. But while all small children have accidents, not all of these accidents result in injuries.

This chapter describes:

- some of the sources of data on child accidents at home, school and play and what these sources tell us about the incidence and prevalence of accidents, the children who have them, where they happen, and when they happen;
- the shortcomings of the data described above. What do they not tell us? What do they obscure? And what kinds of data would tell us more? This section of the chapter will look at whether data on accidents and injuries are useful in telling us anything about the risk to which children are exposed.

In summary, this chapter looks at the some of the patterns of accidents which occur in the home, outside at play or whilst at school. Accidents are the major source of mortality and an important cause of morbidity in the young. For example, as Figure 4.1 shows, nearly a quarter of deaths in the under 5s result from accidents, the great majority occurring in the home. In older children, accident rates are even higher, accounting for over a third of all deaths among 5–14 year olds. However, a change in accident patterns takes place, with older children experiencing a progressively larger number of accidents outside the home, primarily on the roads.

We shall examine these accident patterns, considering both the types of accidents that predominate at different ages, and the factors that seem to give rise to them. Data will be used to illustrate the influence of social, family and environmental factors and attention will also be given to

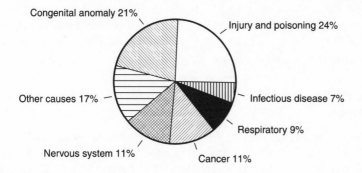

Figure 4.1(a) Causes of death age 1–4 years, UK 1990
Source: Office of Population Censuses and Surveys (OPCS) DH2/17, DH6/4; RG Scotland 1990; RG N. Ireland 1991
Note: Total 1163 deaths

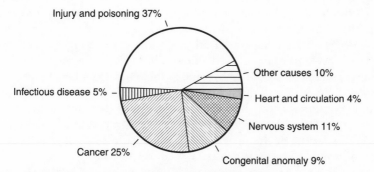

Figure 4.1(b) Causes of death age 5–9 years, UK 1990
Source: OPCS DH2/17, DH6/4; RG Scotland 1990; RG N. Ireland 1991
Note: Total 619 deaths

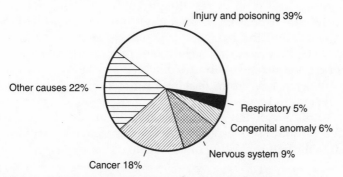

Figure 4.1(c) Causes of death age 10–14 years, UK 1990
Source: OPCS DH2/17, DH6/4; RG Scotland 1990; RG N. Ireland 1991
Note: Total 679 deaths

factors intrinsic to the child (age, sex, ethnicity, stage of development and so on). The aim is to build an overall picture of accidents resulting in death or injury as a prelude to the following chapter which examines accident prevention strategies.

SOURCES OF DATA ON CHILD ACCIDENTS AT HOME, SCHOOL AND PLAY

'Accident' has a wide range of meanings. Events ranging from a small child being unable to reach the lavatory in time, to the pushing and shoving resulting in playground injury: 'But it was an accident . . .'; from a cup of milk being spilt to a child being mown down by a speeding drunken driver are all referred to as accidents. The word 'accident' gives a sense that these things happen by chance. That nothing can be done about them. That they are as random as the fall of the dice.

But an examination of data on those accidents which result in injury or death shows that accidents do not happen at random at all. There are very clear patterns of age, sex and social class. Some parts of the country have much higher accident rates than others, and some countries have much higher (or lower) rates of accidents than others, even within Europe.

Some accidents result in death, some in lifelong or longlasting disability. Some result in serious injury from which the child makes a complete recovery. Some result in the kind of injury which entails a trip to the Accident and Emergency Department, or to the general practitioner's surgery, the dentist or the pharmacist. Others result in a slight injury – a scratch, a bruise, a bump or a graze which can be dealt with in the home, or by a hug and reassurance from dad or mum. Some accidents may result in no injury at all. Sometimes, an accident which seems inevitable is averted either by the child or someone else. Some dangerous places are 'accidents waiting to happen', but they have not happened, or not yet.

The more serious the injury resulting from the accident, on the whole, the better the data we have. It is important to remind ourselves that we are not talking about the seriousness or otherwise of the *accident* itself. The same set of circumstances: a child putting a knitting needle into an electric socket, for instance – 'the accident' – may result in death, serious injury resulting in long-term disability, serious injury from which the child recovers, slight injury, no injury, a 'near-miss' or an averted accident. Factors completely external to the child and the family situation: safety electrical sockets for instance, with on/off switches, are likely to be influential in the natural history of the accident process.

ACCIDENTS RESULTING IN DEATH

Our fullest data on accidents are those relating to accidents which result in death. In the UK, registration systems for death are well developed (Nissel, 1987). Although there may occasionally be some 'fuzziness' round the edges of whether a particular sudden child death is defined as an accident – some suicides and murders may be miscategorised in either direction, for instance – data on accidental death are relatively complete in respect of numbers of deaths, place of death, and age and sex of the child concerned.

Sources of data on deaths from home and other accidents in the UK include:

- Reports from the Registrar General for England and Wales, e.g:

  - OPCS DH1 Mortality statistics: surveillance
  - OPCS DH2 Mortality statistics: cause
  - OPCS DH6 Mortality statistics: childhood

- Annual Reports from the Registrar General for Scotland
- Annual Reports from the Registrar General for Northern Ireland
- Data produced by the Department of Trade and Industry (DTI)

  - the Home Accident Deaths Database (HADD) is particularly concerned to identify the sorts of products associated with deaths in the home in order to consider preventive measures

There are other sources of data on road traffic accidents, dealt with elsewhere in this book. What do these data show?

After the age of 12 months, injuries following an accident are the largest single cause of death to children and young adults in the United Kingdom, with accidental death rates in Scotland and Northern Ireland even higher than those in England and Wales, as Figure 4.2 demonstrates (CAPT, 1989; Woodroffe et al., 1993).

Individual and social characteristics

At every age, boys are more likely to die in accidents than girls. While in older teenagers, where the difference is most pronounced, it is not difficult to speculate on differences in risk taking behaviour, particularly in driving, motorcycling and riskier sports, it is less easy to explain the higher mortality rate of boys under 12 months, under 5 years, or under 10 years shown in Figure 4.3 (Woodroffe et al., 1993). These differences do not seem to be entirely explicable in terms of differences in exposure to risk (Rivara et al., 1982). They may be partly due to differences in behaviour, which are at least in part learned and have been shown in children as young as 1 year old (Maccoby and Jacklin, 1974).

There is a very steep social class gradient in child accident deaths – indeed the steepest social class gradient for any cause of death

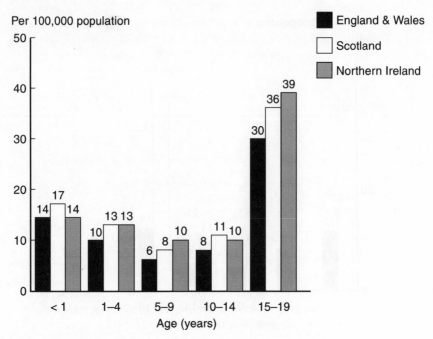

Figure 4.2 Mortality from injuries: age and country, UK 1987–90

Source: OPCS DH2; RG Scotland 1992; RG N. Ireland 1992

(Townsend and Davidson, 1988). Poor children are more likely to die in an accident – and very substantially more likely to die in a fire. This social class gradient is likely to account in large part for the the regional variations in accidents. In a study of 255 fatal childhood accidents from head injury for instance, a 15-fold difference in mortality was observed between local authority wards with the best and the worst deprivation indices (Sharples *et al.*, 1990).

Types of accident resulting in death

In the under 5s, most fatal accidents to children happen in the home. In the over 5s, by far the majority of fatal accidents to children and young people happen on the roads. It does not need a sophisticated epidemiological analysis to demonstrate why this is so. Most children under the age of 5 spend most of their time in the home. They do not travel in vehicles to the same extent as older children, and they are less likely to be unsupervised in the street.

Leaving on one side road accidents, which are discussed in detail elsewhere, fatal accidents to children in the home are most likely to be as

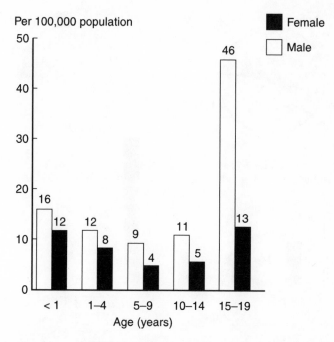

Per 100,000 population

Figure 4.3 Mortality from injuries: age and sex, England and Wales 1987–90
Source: OPCS DH2

a result of burns and scalds, followed by suffocation, drowning, falls and poisoning, as illustrated in Figure 4.4. Accidents in other places (again leaving the roads to one side) are most likely to be drownings, followed by falls.

Trends in child accidental deaths

Firstly, although there has been a fall in the number of children killed in accidents in England and Wales since the 1950s, Figure 4.5 shows that the fall in accidents has not been as steep as the fall in other causes of death for children and young people. It is because of the fall in these other causes of death that child accidents have become the most important single cause of child death. While mortality rates from measles, whooping cough, tuberculosis and pneumonia have plummeted since the turn of the century, and there has been a small fall in mortality from child cancer, accident death rates to children and young people have declined less dramatically. It is difficult to know whether the decline has been due to better preventive methods, better medical and surgical care once an

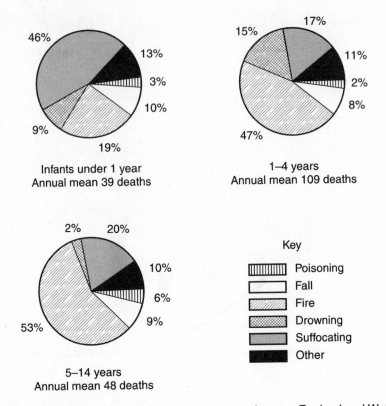

Infants under 1 year
Annual mean 39 deaths

1–4 years
Annual mean 109 deaths

5–14 years
Annual mean 48 deaths

Key

||||||| Poisoning

☐ Fall

▧ Fire

▨ Drowning

▤ Suffocating

■ Other

Figure 4.4 Deaths from accidents at home: age and cause, England and Wales 1987–90

Source: OPCS DH4, ICD E850-949, excluding those outside the home

accident has taken place, or children and their families being exposed to less risk through greater vigilance.

Data on child accident deaths worth further exploration

A fund of data on child accident deaths is available through the records of the coroner or the procurator fiscal's office. While much child accident death data refers simply to the cause of death, the type of accident, and the age and sex of the child, the coroner will frequently be a much richer source of data, exploring the antecedents of the accident as well as the consequences. In her study of coroners' records of child accident deaths, Levene (1991), while pointing out gaps in data in coroners' records, suggests that cooperative coroners can contribute to child safety as their records are rich in information about accidents:

Rate per million living

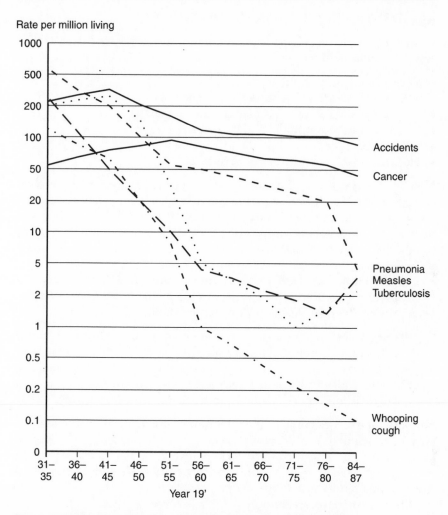

Figure 4.5 Mortality rates from selected causes for children aged 1–14,
England and Wales 1931–87 (rates per million population)

Source: OPCS. Deaths by cause. Quarterly Monitors DH2 88/3, 1988; Child Accident
Prevention Trust, 1989

There was considerable information in the records that did allow
suggestions for prevention to be made. Coroners could make this
information available at a local level where it could inform local
accident prevention groups and community health strategies. It could
contribute to a national database on accidental death (Levene 1991:
1241).

ACCIDENTS RESULTING IN NON-FATAL INJURY

Sources of data on accidents resulting in non-fatal injury at home, at play and in schools include:

- The General Household Survey (GHS)
- The Home Accident Surveillance Scheme (HASS)
- The Leisure Accident Surveillance Scheme (LASS)
- Local authority or school accident records
- GP records
- Hospital admission or treatment records

None of these sources of data provides a perfect picture of those child accidents which result in injury but not death. Data on injury or hospital admission are far more volatile than data on deaths. While the number of deaths which go totally unrecorded in the UK is very small, and the number wrongly recorded to an accidental cause also likely to be small, there are many causes of inaccuracy in data relating to non-fatal injury.

It is likely that the majority of accidents resulting in a severe injury will be brought to the attention of a doctor or hospital, but we know that this is not always the case. As others have pointed out:

> reliance on either attendance at a hospital accident and emergency department, or admission to hospital subsequent to an accident introduces a potentially serious bias . . . Both the action of seeking medical attention, and the decision to admit to hospital are influenced by a variety of factors other than the injury itself. (Stewart-Brown *et al.*, 1986)

Once an injury does come to the attention of the medical profession, the way in which it is recorded, and the accuracy of recording, will depend very much on local factors. Records kept by GPs and hospitals are naturally likely to have more information on the injury itself, and the treatment given, than on the cause of the injury.

Other methods of recording, which involve recall by a parent, or possibly a child, have been shown to be accurate (Agass *et al.*, 1990), but these data, and many *ad hoc* local studies, are not normally aggregated on a national basis. From the point of accident prevention, this is not necessarily a grave problem. Much accident prevention, as will be argued in the next chapter, can most usefully be based on very local data. But many decisions on resource allocation to injury prevention depend on the availability of reliable national and regional data.

Numbers and severity

Something in the order of 120,000 children annually are admitted to hospitals in England and Wales following an accident and about 2 million are treated in an Accident and Emergency department (CAPT, 1989). During the period 1987–9, 19 per cent of 0–4 year olds and 15 per cent of 5–15 year olds consulted their family doctor following an accident (Woodroffe *et al.*, 1993).

Data on the long term consequences of accidents are difficult to access, but one study suggests that about 3 per cent of children under the age of 15 admitted to hospital after an accident have a permanent disability as a consequence of the accident (Avery and Gibbs, 1985). Unpublished data from the National Child Development Survey (NCDS) suggests an even more worrying pattern. This large birth cohort study indicates that, for 16–23 year olds, a permanent disability results from at least 9 per cent of accidents resulting in admission to hospital, and 2 per cent of those treated in an Accident and Emergency department (M. Barker and C. Power, unpublished data in Woodroffe *et al.*, 1993: 113).

Individual and social characteristics

We know less about the social class composition of people who are injured in accidents than we do about people who die from accidents. However, a number of studies have shown non-fatal accidents to be related to family size (the larger the family, the more likely an accident); overcrowded accommodation; housing tenure (accidents are more common in council housing); unemployed fathers and low level of parental education (Wadsworth, 1983; Pless *et al.*, 1989). The main correlates of child accidents are also indicators of social deprivation.

But there is also a body of work on the psychological and psycho-social correlates of child accidents. Brown and Davidson (1978) related child accidents to maternal depression. Personality traits some researchers have found to be associated with accidents include anxiety, instability, hyperactivity, clumsiness and aggression (Sibert and Newcombe, 1977; Bijur *et al.*, 1986; Gilberg, 1987). We should bear in mind that all these observations do is *describe* the social characteristics of children having accidents or their parents, not explain why they have them, far less prevent them.

Type of accident

There are differences in the patterns of the type of accident resulting in a non-fatal injury, and those resulting in death. While deaths from fire account for 12 per cent of accidental deaths of under ones, 25 per cent of accidental deaths of 1–4 year olds, 11 per cent of 5–9 year olds and 3 per cent of 10–14 year olds, burns represent only 6 per cent of injuries presenting at an Accident and Emergency department for 0–4 year olds and 3 per cent for 5–14 year olds. The most common non-fatal accidents (apart from road accidents) needing hospital treatment are falls, followed among

0–4 year olds by being struck by an object, the presence of a foreign body, poisoning, cuts and bites. For older children and young people, the pattern is falls, followed by being struck, cuts, foreign body, bites, burns and poisoning (Woodroffe *et al.*, 1993).

Location of accident

Most non-fatal accidents to children and young people happen either on the road, involving a vehicle, or at home. For those that do not, the majority still happen in streets or parking areas. For many children, their playspace is the street or the carpark. The next most common location is schools and nurseries, followed by recreational areas, sports facilities and industrial worksites or farms. These accidents are reported through the Leisure Accidents Surveillance Scheme (LASS), conducted by the Department of Trade and Industry. Many schoolchildren, presumably, would find it ironical that school accidents are included in the leisure accidents scheme.

An excellent and underused source of data on (usually) non-fatal accidents are the records of school accidents. These are normally kept for administrative (insurance) reasons, which means that coverage is very good, but they tend not to be analysed in aggregate. Because the records are normally kept by non-medical personnel (school secretaries, helpers, or teachers), there tends to be a concentration on the hazardous event as well as the injury. In medical records on the other hand, there is not surprisingly a far greater concentration on the injuries which follow the accident than the circumstances preceding it. In terms of preventing accidents, information on the antecedents of the accidents – what was going on at the time, when and where, are rather more likely to be helpful in preventing recurrences than describing the injuries following an accident. The data described in Figure 4.6 shows where accidents occur in Glasgow primary and secondary schools (Roberts *et al.*, 1992a; CAPT and Roberts, 1993). The following chapter describes the ways in which data like these can be used in accident prevention schemes at a very local level.

NEAR-MISSES, AVERTED ACCIDENTS AND ACCIDENTS WHICH DO NOT RESULT IN AN INJURY REQUIRING MEDICAL ATTENTION

If we think of accidents in terms of a triangle with a relatively small number of deaths at the apex, the wide base of the triangle, the events which occur most often, will be those accidents which do not require an undertaker, long- or short-term hospitalisation or even a trip to the Accident and Emergency department. These are the 'near-misses': the child who escapes serious injury because the tile which falls off the school

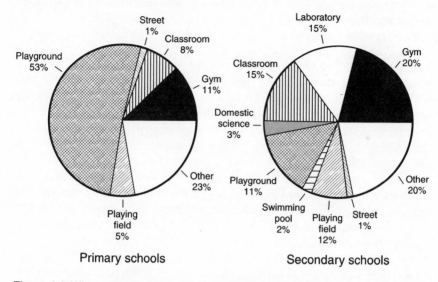

Figure 4.6 Where accidents happen in schools in Glasgow

Source: Strathclyde Regional Council internal accident report forms, January to June 1989 and 1991 (charts based on 546 accidents in primary schools and 635 accidents in secondary schools)

roof doesn't fall off at playtime, or the iron pulled off the ironing board does not make contact with the child. They are also the averted accidents: the child who escapes being mown down by the car or lorry because miraculously, although the vehicle is speeding, the driver manages to swerve or brake at the last moment. They are the accidents where a child falls off the scaffolding erected to do something about the fabric of the building, or crawls through the nifty gap in the balcony in the council flat, and walks away without a scratch.

Not all accidents end in tears, although all dangerous events, people and places are a health hazard in terms of anxiety to parents and carers, and restriction on the lives of children.

This pool of largely unanalysed data on the accidents which don't happen could be a valuable tool in preventing accidents. In high risk activities such as anaesthetics and aviation, 'near-misses' form important data in the formulation of safety policies. The accidents waiting to happen, or barely averted, are the ones we can avoid in future. Just as crime has been largely 'designed out' of some housing estates, with door-phones, breaking up the 'walkways in the skies', improving lighting, and changing housing allocation policies, there is ample scope for 'designing out' many accidents to children, by using the knowledge of local people on dangerous places and events. This is discussed in more detail in the following chapter.

But how do you collect data on accidents which don't happen, or which do happen and don't result in injury, or which result in injury, but not of the sort that will find its way into official statistics, because it is treated at home or by the GP? These kind of data are rarely collected, and when they are, are collected through small local surveys. Two examples are from Glasgow studies (CAPT and Roberts, 1993; Roberts *et al.*, 1992a; Roberts *et al.*, 1995). In a study of the way in which parents keep their children safe in unsafe surroundings we asked a number of questions touching on this.

Almost a third of the parents in the community could recall a serious accident which their child had had which had not resulted in injury. The same number could think of other examples in their community where dangerous things had happened to children, not necessarily their own, without their getting hurt.

We asked: 'Sometimes, we can see a child about to do something really dangerous, and we are able to stop it at the last minute; or a child runs out into the road, but the motorist is able to avoid her at the last minute. We're thinking here about near-misses, and wonder if you can think of any near-misses your own children have had?'

Almost half of the parents we interviewed could think of such an incident; moreover 60 per cent – particularly parents of older children – were sure that there were other near-misses of which they were blissfully unaware (Roberts *et al.*, 1995).

A further series of questions allowed us to look at the accident in more detail. We asked where the (near) accident had happened, what the child had been doing at the time, what went wrong, how the accident was avoided, and any precautions or changes made since. Not surprisingly, many parents used these 'near-misses' to inform their own safety behaviour:

> A nearly accident, I think you have a nearly accident every day really as far as the kids are concerned – y'know, they've done this and you've stopped them, nearly went near this . . . or you maybe sense that there's something they're doing.'

> 'It's when you see them nearly doing something that you realize that that's the danger or this is the danger . . . That's how you get experience . . . by the things they nearly do and don't do – sometimes the things they do.' (Roberts *et al.*, 1992b)

About a quarter of parents in the community reported at least one accident to a child or children in the week before they were questioned which resulted in an injury which was treated at home. A substantial minority reported several.

In the Glasgow school study (CAPT and Roberts, 1993), questions were again asked about accidents which had not quite happened. Children were asked not only about accidents which had happened at school, or on the way to or from school, but also accidents which had nearly happened at school or on the journey. These accidents which had not quite occurred were a rich source of data particularly on road traffic accidents, where children characterised adult driver behaviour as perverse, unpredictable, and generally substandard, as we shall see in the following chapter.

As much is obscured as is revealed by the data on child accidents. Statistical data are themselves social constructs, and are collected for a variety of different purposes. Since much data on accidents and injuries is kept largely for administrative purposes, it is hardly surprising that the quality and extent of data which would be most useful for preventing accidents are largely missing.

Official data on accidents are also interesting in that they tend to tell us more about the victim of the accident (his or her behaviour, age, and state of health) than about the person or set of events on the other side of the accident. We therefore know more about the unpredictability and behaviour patterns of children than we do about the unpredictability and behaviour patterns of motorists, designers of playgrounds and town planners.

In addition, we know a good deal more about the numerator in accident data – the children who do have accidents, than the denominator – the whole population of children. This makes it very difficult to understand issues like the level of risk to which children are exposed. This uncollected data may also help to explain why there are so few accidents, for instance, in a particular playground which all the mothers and children on a particular estate 'know' is dangerous. It may simply be that it is a place which is not used, is 'banned' or where, because the dangers are known, extra precautions are exercised.

This chapter has given examples of some of the data we have, and some of the data we do not have, which shed light on child accidents at home, at school and at play. For all that they are partial and incomplete, the data do tell us important things about accidents, the most important being that accidents do not happen at random. They are not entirely unpredictable, and there is a steep social class gradient, with the poorest children being at the greatest risk of an accident.

One source of data on accidents only touched on here, but which will be explored in more detail in the next chapter, is the huge reservoir of detailed and reliable data which ordinary children and families have about the accident risks in their own environments and their own lives, and the ways in which these data are used – sometimes imperfectly – to prevent accidents.

REFERENCES

Agass, M., Mant, D., Fuller, A., Coulter, A. and Jones, L. (1990) 'Childhood accidents: a practice survey using general practitioners' records and parental reports', *British Journal of General Practice* 40, 334: 202–5.

Avery, J. G. and Gibbs, B. (1985) 'Long term disability following accidents in childhood', in *Proceedings of Symposium on Accidents in Childhood*, Occasional paper no. 7, 27–39, London: Child Accident Prevention Trust.

Bijur, P., Stewart-Brown, S. and Butler, N. (1986) 'Child behaviour and accidental injury in 11,966 pre-school children', *American Journal of Diseases of Children* 140: 492–587.

Brown, G. and Davidson, S. (1978) 'Social class, psychiatric disorder of mother and accidents to children', *Lancet* 1: 8060: 378–80.

Child Accident Prevention Trust (CAPT) (1989) *Basic Principles of Child Accident Prevention: A Guide to Action*, London: Child Accident Prevention Trust

CAPT and Roberts, H. (1993) *A Safe School Is No Accident*, London: Child Accident Prevention Trust.

Gilberg, C. (1987) 'The relationship of accidents to intelligence, personality and handicap', in R. Berfenstam, H. Jackson and B. Eriksson (eds) *The Healthy Community: Child Safety as a part of Health Promotion Activities*, Stockholm: Folksam.

Levene, S. (1991) 'Coroners' records of accidental deaths', *Archives of Disease in Childhood* 66: 1239–41.

Maccoby, E. and Jacklin, C. (1974) *The Psychology of Sex Differences*, Stanford: Stanford University Press.

Nissel, M. (1987) *People Count: A History of the General Register Office*, London: HMSO.

Pless, I. B., Peckham, C. S. and Power, C. (1989) 'Predicting traffic injuries in childhood: a cohort analysis', *Journal of Paediatrics* 115, 6: 932–8.

Rivara, F. P., Bergman, A. B., LoGerfo, J. P. and Weiss, N. S. (1982) 'Epidemiology of childhood injuries: sex differences in injury rates', *American Journal of Diseases of Children* 136: 502–6.

Roberts, H., McLoone, P. and Balendra, R. (1992a) 'Report to the trustees of the Nuffield Foundation on school accidents in Glasgow: a public health approach', unpublished.

Roberts, H., Smith, S. J. and Lloyd, M. (1992b) 'Safety as a social value: a community approach', in S. Scott, G. Williams, S. Platt and H. Thomas (eds) *Private Risks and Public Dangers*, Aldershot: Avebury.

Roberts, H., Smith, S. J. and Bryce, C. (1995) *Children at Risk? Safety as a Social Value*, Milton Keynes: Open University Press.

Sharples, P. M., Storey, A., Aynsley Green, A. and Eyre, J. A. (1990) 'Causes of fatal childhood accidents involving head injury in Northern region, 1979–86', *British Medical Journal* 301: 1193–7.

Sibert, J. and Newcombe, R. G. (1977) 'Accidental ingestion of poisons and child personality', *Postgraduate Medical Journal* 53: 254–6.

Stewart-Brown, S., Peters, T. J., Godling, J. and Bijur, P. (1986) 'Case definition in childhood accident studies: a vital factor in determining results', *International Journal of Epidemiology* 15, 3: 352–9.

Townsend, P. and Davidson, N. (1988) *The Black Report*, Harmondsworth: Penguin.

Wadsworth, J., Burnell, I. and Butler, N. (1983) 'Family type and accidents in pre-school children', *Journal of Epidemiology and Community Health* 37: 100–104.

Woodroffe, C., Glickman, M., Barker, M. and Power, C. (1993) *Children, Teenagers and Health: the Key Data*, Milton Keynes: Open University Press.

Chapter 5

Intervening to prevent accidents

Helen Roberts

The previous chapter showed that a major problem with accident data (or more properly, injury data) is that it largely excludes all those accidents treated in Accident and Emergency departments, at home, or by general practitioners and dentists. Injury data thus underestimate the true incidence, leaving an 'iceberg' of unreported events that are not well understood. The incidence and patterning of 'near-misses' are not recorded either, nor do we have any idea of the strategies that parents or children routinely adopt to keep themselves and their families safe.

A number of other chapters refer to the weighty child protection procedures, intended to protect children from violent injuries and death in the private sphere of the home, yet those whose duty it is to protect children have not expended the same energy on the public sphere: the dangers children face from poor housing, poor playspaces and an environment which is generally hostile to children. While the rhetoric of the social welfare world is 'empowerment,' the preferred mode of operation continues to be individually or family based interventions, with a focus on putting right parental deficits. This chapter will suggest that there are other ways of keeping children safe which could be tried and subjected to the kinds of rigorous evaluation so frequently lacking in studies of health promotion.

Childhood accidents are a major health problem. They have been recognised as such in important policy and strategy documents (DoH, 1992; NHSME, 1992; Towner et al., 1993) and there is currently a climate in which accident prevention is seen as crucial in improving the health of the nation. But what do we know about the kinds of things we need to do in order to prevent child accidents at home, at school and at play? And looking at the range of things which could be done, how sure are we that the preventive interventions we choose are effective? How do we know whether our well intentioned attempts to reduce childhood accidents are having the desired effect? Is it possible there might be some unintended adverse effects from trying to prevent children's accidents? Might we make children more fearful, for instance, in much the same way as a focus on crime has made fear of crime a problem in its own right. Might we inadvertently stifle children's sense of adventure or discourage children's independence? We already know that many more children are driven by car to primary school than was the case twenty years ago (Hillman *et al.*, 1990) and that this not only restricts the mobility of the children chauffeured to school, but it also increases the risk to children who walk. And it not only increases their risk of a road traffic accident, but also increases their risk from traffic pollution.

Many interventions in children's lives, accident prevention among them, are seen as self-evidently a good thing. As Stone (1989: 891) has pointed out: 'Health education is cheap, generally uncontroversial and safe: if it works, politicians take the credit, and if it does not, the target population takes the blame.' Critical scrutiny of the effectiveness of accident prevention measures has until recently been viewed askance. What could possibly be wrong with putting a leaflet into every child's hand before the summer holiday telling them of some of the dangers of swimming? Surely they need to be informed; and won't having this information help them to do the right thing?

Sadly, we know that the links between knowledge, attitudes and behaviour are by no means straightforward. If they were, it is unlikely that anyone would smoke, take drugs, or have unprotected sex. But the standard reaction to this self-evident truth has frequently been to try and find better ways of communicating the message, or to blame the delinquent recipients of health education messages for not gratefully seizing on the information they are given. For despite the lack of corroborating evidence, health education in its simplest knowledge transfer from 'experts' to lay people continues to be seen as a major plank of child accident prevention.

The recommendations of The Health of the Nation Focus Groups, for instance, suggest that purchasing negotiations and NHS contracts for acute services require 'health promotion material relating to accident prevention to be available in the A & E department and other appropriate locations. This material should, where appropriate, be available in languages other than English'. For community services, a recommendation is to: 'require that health promotion material relating to accident prevention is available in community clinics and other appropriate locations. This material should, where appropriate, be available in languages other than English' (NHSME, 1992: 43).

Health promotion materials are not the most expensive of health interventions. They are far less expensive for instance, than surgical intervention in a tertiary centre of excellence, trying to put right the consequences of an accident, but are they as effective? The recommendation that health education materials be available at all health outlets, suggests a very considerable volume of printed material. Translating health promotion materials is a specialised task, and having these materials available in other languages presupposes considerable development work, since translation of these kinds of materials involves not simply a technical task, but a sensitive understanding of cultural patterns and mores. One is therefore talking about considerable expenditure. Do we have good evidence that this material will significantly benefit people other than those who write the material, and those who print it?

Surprisingly enough, we do not. Ampofo-Boateng and Thomson's (1989) important review of current approaches to child pedestrian accidents in the UK suggests that verbal instructions to children can be hazardous when used in isolation. Behavioural changes advocated by posters and other printed material are rarely evaluated (Gerber *et al.*, 1977), but such evidence as there is suggests that they are not effective. While this material may increase children's knowledge, it does not readily transfer to behaviour (Schioldborg, 1976). Ampofo-Boateng and Thomson have drawn attention to the difficulties children face in built up areas in following injunctions to make sure no cars are coming before crossing the road, or never to cross between parked cars. Parents and children may face similar problems when addressing issues of safety in the home, at play and at school. While the exhortation to parents never to leave children alone in the home is self-evidently wise, it fails to address the context in which a number of health promoting childcare tasks, including feeding, cleaning, and earning, compete for priority in the majority of households. Health promotion advice which addresses the *content* of health behaviour outside the *context* in which that behaviour takes place is unlikely to succeed. Posters available until recently from a health promotion source showed two mothers outside a school exhorting: 'Meet them: don't let them die on the roads.' Other educational material suggests that:

- *Accidents may happen when adults are*:

  - Under stress
  - Less alert – this may be due to tiredness, worry etc.

- To children who are:

  - Overprotected
  - Underprotected
  - Not supervised
  - Angry
  - Tired
  - Under stress
  - Impulsive
  - Showing off

While this may well be true, these characteristics are so widely found among parents and children that they practically rehearse the condition of much of parenthood, and some of childhood. They are therefore unhelpful as diagnostic tools. What preventive behaviour might stem from this? The same material suggests:

Reduce the risks by:
  Setting a good example
  Making sure the home and garden are as safe as possible
  Teaching children to be aware of dangers and how to cope with them
  Never leaving them on their own
  Buying toys and equipment that are safety approved and checked.

While this health promotion advice is no doubt well-meaning, and is eminently sensible, how practical is it for a family living in poverty three floors above the green where washing is hung; where money for toys is short; where parents are living in bed and breakfast accommodation and are faced with the choice of leaving children locked in their room, or taking them to a kitchen two floors away which is shared with other families and has sub-optimal safety equipment?

 In any case, a number of studies suggests that parental knowledge of home accidents, and risks to children, is high (Colver et al., 1982; Roberts, 1991; Roberts et al., 1992, 1993a, 1993b) and that children, even of primary school age, are very aware of risks in their own school environments (CAPT and Roberts, 1993). Such health education programmes as have been evaluated have been disappointing (Schlesinger, 1966) or have concentrated on inappropriate outcome measures. There is little point in knowing that every health visitor working in a certain area has put a leaflet into the hand of every mother of an under five, and given personalised advice, if we do not know whether the accident rate is reduced, increased or unchanged, as a result. Moreover, we also need to know of other health gains or losses. Is maternal anxiety reduced or increased by health education interventions? If it is increased, we know that parental stress is a precipitating factor for child accidents. Certainly, many of the parents interviewed in the Corkerhill study, while in many cases valuing health visitor advice, were at best less than convinced, and at worst irritated by exhortation on safety matters:

> you get really depressed, and think about the things your children should have. You're told all the time, you know, you get these millions of books when you have a baby, and all this equipment you should have, and it can end up [with you thinking], 'I'm no' bringing my child up properly,' . . . and it just adds to all the other stresses you've got.
>
> (Roberts et al., 1992: 197–8)

Given then that there is still a great deal to know about the effectiveness of accident prevention, what might be the 'best buys' in preventing accidents in the home, in schools and in the wider environment? What sorts of methods of preventing accidents seem most likely to meet with a degree of success? If straightforward health education in the form of posters, leaflets and exhortation does seem to offer helpful results in terms of reduced accidents and more general health gains, what does look promising?

KEEPING CHILDREN SAFE AT HOME, SCHOOL AND IN THE WIDER ENVIRONMENT

The following key issues can be identified as pointers for different groups of practitioners:

Accurate data on accidents and 'near-misses'

As the previous chapter argues, current data on the prevalence of accidents are heavily biased, as they rely mainly on deaths and hospital admissions, whereas many childhood accidents are treated by parents, by GPs or dentists, or in Accident and Emergency departments. As every parent knows, exactly the same sequence of events can have tragic, serious, minor or no consequences. As others have pointed out, the accidents which are recorded refer to the dangerous places, events and behaviours which children don't get away with. It has long been recognised in other fields, for instance accidents at work, anaesthetic accidents and aviation accidents that for the effective prevention of accidents, we need data on the near-misses and the minor accidents, as well as the tragedies, in order to develop effective safety strategies. *Improved information on accidents and their distribution, including accidents at the most local level, is required if effective public health prevention policies are to be formulated.*

Practical steps might include the following.

At a national level

- For the Department of Health: to ensure a national system of data collection on child accidents so that in comparing one region with another, one is comparing like with like. The information collected should refer to events before the accident (the precipitants) as well as the sequelae. A 'pick list' of precipitating factors should be capable of identifying environmental, social and institutional factors, e.g. traffic lights out of order; no supervision in playground; as well as individual behavioural factors, e.g. mother hanging out washing while child is momentarily alone.

At a regional and local level

- For the Director of Public Health: to ensure that adequate information systems are in place.
- For public health staff to look at coroners' records with a view to exploring at a local level which deaths may have been preventable, and how they may have been prevented.
- For health visitors, as well as imparting health education information, to collect health education material from parents on the ways in which they keep children safe in unsafe environments; on near misses, and on averted accidents.
- For school nurses or others with access to school accident data to collate data on accidents within particular schools, with a view to using this to work with the school, with children and with parents on effective accident prevention (for methods of doing this, see CAPT and Roberts, 1993).

How parents keep their children safe

More effort should be spent on identifying parents' and children's own perceptions of hazards. These perspectives help identify the strategies that parents currently take to protect their children, and help identify problem areas. Along with colleagues with whom I have worked closely, and others active in health promotion (Roberts *et al.*, 1993a; Popay and Williams, 1994), I believe that people who live in a particular environment (Roberts *et al.*, 1995), and are daily engaged in the task of looking after children, are better placed, on the whole, than are health and social welfare professionals to be aware of, and responsive to, the risks in their own environments. The interesting question in child accident prevention is not 'Why are there so many child accidents?' but 'Why, given the dangers of the environment in which most children grow up, are there so few?' Little is known about the strategies which parents and children routinely incorporate into the structure of their everyday lives to keep themselves and those for whom they are responsible safe. Such strategies need to be better understood. We need to know not only what they are, but why they sometimes fail, or fail to be implemented. What are the pressure points which cause parents to drop well honed safety strategies, and what protective mechanisms might be built in to prevent this happening? *Professionals should attempt to build on the 'lay knowledge' of ordinary people and communities.* Effective health promotion, including the prevention of accidents, is likely to happen when we draw on the strengths and abilities which ordinary people already have in negotiating their everyday lives, and learning from these. Ordinary children and their families, after all, successfully avoid accidents every day. We should learn both from their successes, and from the lessons to be learned when their strategies fail.

Practical steps might include the following.

At a national level

- For the Health Education Authority (England and Wales) and the Health Education Boards (Scotland and Northern Ireland) to encourage the collection of data on lay expertise, in order for more health education material to be firmly grounded in the realities of the lives of those at whom the education is aimed. (Articles in Popay and Williams, 1994, give examples of ways in which this might operate.)

At a regional and local level

- For Departments of Public Health, Departments of Health Promotion and Health Visitors to use local data as described in the previous section to work with local communities drawing on their expertise and knowledge, to use both quantitative and qualitative data to build preventive strategies embedded at the local level.

Designing for safety

Design and engineering play an important part in accident prevention. The most effective preventive measures are frequently the 'passive' ones, the ones to which we barely need to give a second thought. These might include on/off switches on electrical sockets, child resistant containers for medicines and household poisons, and devices which turn off electrical appliances once they get too hot.

There is some evidence which points to the ways in which accidents can be designed out of streets and roads. The *woonerven* in the Netherlands, and the separation of children from traffic in some areas in the Nordic countries fall into the subject matter of another chapter. But can accidents be designed out of children's homes, out of their playspaces or out of their schools and nurseries? The answer is that entirely designing out accidents is not only impossible, but is probably not even desirable. A degree of risk, and opportunities to take risks are part of the normal development of every child. For a toddler, standing up in her cot, or walking across the room involves some risk. And not only do children need to take some risks in order to develop new abilities and skills: taking risks can be enjoyable, as every Scottish mountain climber knows. The sense of achievement a child may have from climbing a tree, coming down a slide for the first time, or jumping over a ditch are not necessarily risks we would want to 'design out'. There is a degree of risk, and children do get hurt, and occasionally get hurt badly from engaging in these activities, but responsible adults (and responsible children, at the stage where children can reasonably be responsible for some of their own safety decisions), may feel that a life entirely without risk is a dull one. The question of 'designing out' some domestic and school dangers is rather different. There is quite enough scope for excitement in the home and at school without needing to add to it with balconies which have gaps a child can crawl through, electric sockets with no on / off switch or a lack of smoke alarms. Estate managers, health promotion staff and others need to work closely with those whose lives make them experts on the design failures which result in accidents, to see which accidents could be 'designed out'. There are a number of examples, in the King's Cross area of London for instance, where a good deal of drugs related crime, has been 'designed out' of the built environment through effective collaboration between a number of agencies and residents.

Practical steps might include the following.

At a national level

- For the Department of the Environment and the Department of Transport to look at the human and economic costs of *not* taking a child protection approach to new projects.

At a regional and local level

- For housing and estate managers to work with tenants on safety audits, identifying those unsafe elements in the environments amenable to change. It is frequently possible to identify low cost as well as high cost solutions.

Children's perceptions of risk

Little attention has been paid to the child's own perception of risk. In many situations, children – even young children – are well informed on risk, and are able to identify risks which may not be evident, or seem so important, to adults. Many primary school children for instance, rightly identify the playground and the school lavatories as 'risky' places. Not only are children able, in many cases, to identify risks. They can also make sensible suggestions for ways to reduce those risks. One way of doing this is through promoting school safety. There are materials which enable children to draw on the accident data for their own school, and work on ways of reducing school accidents. This approach has the added benefit that, since schools are relatively closed communities, and normally have excellent accident reporting systems for less serious as well as more serious accidents, there is scope for good measurement of the effects of any programme introduced, with before and after data readily to hand. (Roberts and CAPT, 1993; University of Glasgow Media Services and Roberts, 1992.) Two children in the school accident study described near-misses:

> 'I was skipping down the lane. The green man was on the screen. I went and crossed the road. I was in the middle of the road when this car went through the red light.'

> 'It was the time when I was walking to school and the green man was on and I was walking across and this car went straight through the green man and [I] just moved back in time, otherwise I would have been knocked down.'

These were not isolated incidents, and brought a chorus of recognition in group discussion, together with a rehearsal of children's sense of injustice that grown-ups didn't 'get into trouble' nearly enough when they infringed safety codes. The children would no doubt have had their sense of 'not fair' heightened had they seen a report commissioned by the Central Research Unit of the Scottish Office (MVA, 1989). Entitled: 'Must do better', those primarily identified as needing to do better were child pedestrians, rather than motorists. *A much greater emphasis should be made on identifying what children of different ages think of as dangerous, and to identify the kinds of solutions they offer*.

Practical steps might include the following.

At a national level

- For the Health Education Authorities and Boards to ensure that children's perspectives are included, not only in the 'market testing' of health education material, but also in the generation of knowledge and understanding which underpins the material.
- For the research councils to ensure that children's perspectives and views are better represented in research on safety, and that appropriate methodologies are developed with good ethical standards, given the vulnerability of children to be encouraged to participate in research without fully informed consent.

At a regional and local level

- For health promoters, teachers, school nurses and others to work with children, recognising, as well as their need to be educated, the reservoir of knowledge they frequently have on dangerous places, events, and (sometimes) people.

Using local knowledge

Community based approaches can be set up, where people identify and define local dangers, and suggest solutions. Parents have an intimate familiarity with the distribution of local hazards, and actively employ this knowledge to keep their children safe most of the time. Children have an intimate familiarity with scary places, and places where you might have an accident at school or on the way to or from school. Safety is practised in communities as well as by individuals and in families. Safety, in effect, is a social as well as an individual value. This has been recognised by, for instance, Rochdale local authority, where the Child Accident Prevention Group has commissioned a children's charity, Barnardo's, to work with children and parents in a particular area of the town, Wardleworth, to identify risks, hazards and safety strategies. These will then be built into a plan aimed to reduce child accidents in the area. The most effective community safety plans are likely to be built on healthy alliances, which fully include local adults and children.

Practical steps might include the following.

At a national level

- The Health Education Authority and Boards to consider, on a pilot basis, setting up a number of community safety schemes, building on local knowledge, skills and expertise. Given that we do not have convincing evidence that the production of written accident prevention material, or posters, is effective, such interventions might be funded by a trial in which 'routine health education' campaigns were rigorously compared with community based projects building on lay knowledge, 'matching' communities in advance on deprivation indices, and numbers of recorded accidents.

At a regional and local level

- For local authorities, as part of their Children's Plans, to look carefully at the dangers to children in the public sphere, as well as in the private sphere, and explore ways of building on community approaches to develop a more holistic view of child protection.

CONCLUSIONS

The state of scientific knowledge on child accident prevention currently leaves a good deal to be desired. While the truism that prevention is better than cure has a number of attractions, the fact that prevention can be cheap (or even free) should not necessarily lead us to suspend our critical faculties. In the last few years, a number of critiques from sociology, social policy, political science and public health medicine have challenged the view that prevention should be exempt from the critical scrutiny which should characterise all intervention in health matters (Graham, 1979, 1988, 1991; Freeman, 1992; Stone, 1986; Williams, 1984; Scrabanek, 1990). I have suggested a number of practical steps which individuals and institutions might take to develop accident prevention work. It is important that any such work be properly evaluated to test whether the interventions are doing good, harm, or whether the jury is out.

Meanwhile, not everything done in terms of social welfare needs to be rigorously tested. We can assume, for instance, that some interventions such as adequate food, clothing and shelter are not harmful, and on the contrary, are a good thing. At present, children while occupying a high position in western societies in terms of rhetoric, occupy a rather lower status when it comes to considering the larger policies which may affect their lives. At a family, local, regional and national level, more could be done to take the interests of children, and their views and knowledge seriously. The possibilities of this having unintended adverse side effects are slight.

ACKNOWLEDGEMENTS

The data described in this chapter, and the previous one, are the result of collaboration with a large number of people, whose work I gratefully acknowledge. These are the people of Corkerhill, Glasgow, and in particular, Cathy Rice, Betty Campbell and Walter Morrison; the staff, children and school board of Hillhead Primary School and the Education Department of Strathclyde Region. Susan J. Smith, Carol Bryce, Michelle Lloyd, Margaret Reilly and I worked together on the Corkerhill study, and Hannah Bradby, Tessa Kelly, Rani Balendra, Philip McLoone and I worked together on the school accident study.

REFERENCES

Ampofo-Boateng, K. and Thomson J. A. (1989) 'Child pedestrian accidents: a case for preventive medicine', *Health Education Research* 5: 265–74.
Child Accident Prevention Trust and Roberts, H. (1993) *A Safe School Is No Accident*, London: Child Accident Prevention Trust.
Colver, A. F., Hutchinson, P. J. and Judson, E. C. (1982) 'Promoting children's home safety', *British Medical Journal* 285: 1177–80.
Department of Health (DoH) (1992) *The Health of the Nation: A Strategy for Health in England*, London: HMSO.
Freeman, R. (1992) 'The idea of prevention: a critical review', in S. Scott, G. Williams, S. Platt and H. Thomas (eds) *Private Risks and Public Dangers*, Avebury: Ashgate.
Gerber, D., Huber, O. and Limbourg, M. (1977) *Verkehrserziehung in Vorschulalter*, Cologne: Woolters Nordhoff.

Graham, H. (1979) 'Prevention and health: every mother's business: a comment on child health policies in the seventies', in C. Harris, (ed.) *The Sociology of the Family. New Directions for Britain*, University of Keele, Sociological Review Monograph no. 28.

Graham, H. (1988) 'Child health: mother's heartache', *Maternity Action*, September–October, 36: 6–7.

Graham, H. (1991) 'Looking after yourself and caring for others: policies and patterns in contemporary Britain', paper presented to British Sociological Association annual conference.

Hillman, M., Adams, J. and Whitelegg, J. (1990) *One False Move: A Study of Children's Independent Mobility*, London: Policy Studies Institute.

MVA Consultancy (1989) *'Must Do Better': A Study of Child Pedestrian Accidents and Road Crossing Behaviour in Scotland*, Edinburgh: Central Research Unit Papers, Scottish Office.

National Health Service Management Executive (NHSME) (1992) *The Health of the Nation: First Steps for the NHS*, London: NHSME.

Popay, J. and Williams, G. (1994) *Researching the Public Health*, London: Routledge and Kegan Paul.

Rice, C., Roberts, H., Smith, S.J. and Bryce, C. (1994) 'It's like teaching your child to swim in a pool full of alligators', in J. Popay and G. Williams, *op. cit.*.

Roberts, H. (1991) 'Accident Prevention: Child Protection', *Health Visitor* 64: 219–21.

Roberts, H., Smith, S. J. and Lloyd, M. (1992) 'Safety as a social value: a community approach', in S. Scott, G. Williams, S. Platt and H. Thomas (eds) *Private Risks and Public Dangers*, Aldershot: Avebury Press.

Roberts, H., Smith, S. J. and Bryce, C. (1993a) 'Prevention is better . . .', *Sociology of Health and Illness* 15, 4: 447–63.

Roberts, H., Smith, S. J. and Bryce, C. (1993b) 'Safety as a social value', final report to the Scottish Office Home and Health Department, Glasgow: Public Health Research Unit.

Roberts, H., Smith, S. J. and Bryce, C. (1995) *Children at Risk*, Milton Keynes: Open University Press.

Schioldborg, P. (1976) *Children, Traffic and Traffic Training: An Analysis of a Children's Traffic Club*, Geilo, Norway: International Federation of Pedestrians.

Schlesinger, E. R. (1966) 'A controlled study of health education in accident prevention', *American Journal of Diseases of Children* 3, 490–6.

Scrabanek, P. (1990) 'Why is preventive medicine exempted from ethical constraints?', *Journal of Medical Ethics* 16: 187–90.

Stone, D. (1986) 'The resistible rise of preventive medicine', *Journal of Health Politics, Policy and Law* 11: 671–96.

Stone, D. (1989) 'Upside down prevention', *Health Service Journal* 99, 20 July: 890–1.

Towner, E., Dowswell, T. and Jarvis, S. (1992) *Reducing Childhood Accidents: The Effectiveness of Health Promotion Interventions: A Literature Review*, London: Health Education Authority.

Towner, E., Dowswell, T. and Jarvis, S. (1993) *The Effectiveness of Health Promotion Interventions in the Prevention of Uninentional Childhood Injury: A Review of the Literature*, London: Health Education Authority.

University of Glasgow Media Services and Roberts, H. (1992) *A Safe School is No Accident*, Video and worksheets (which can be freely photocopied) available from University of Glasgow Media Services, 20 Southpark Avenue, Glasgow G12 8LB. Price £20.00 inc VAT and p.&p.

Williams, G. (1984) 'Health promotions – caring concern or slick salesmanship?', *Journal of Medical Ethics* 10: 191–5.

Chapter 6

Child pedestrian accidents: what makes children vulnerable?

James A. Thomson

In the year following publication of this book, around 5,000 child pedestrians will be seriously injured or killed while trying to cross the road and another 15,000 will be 'slightly' injured; that is, they will require medical attention and the circumstances surrounding their injury will have been sufficiently serious to have been recorded by the police. This prediction about future accident rates does not depend on premonition or hours spent poring over astrological charts. It follows from the consistency with which such accidents have occurred in the past, making their prediction in the future as safe a bet as you are ever likely to find. Even within a local area, police officers can often tell with disconcerting accuracy *how many* pedestrian accidents will take place over a given period of time; *where* the accidents are most likely to happen; *when* they will take place; and even *who* is most likely to be involved.

The regularities in the accident pattern from one year to the next and even from one country to the next is astonishing. And yet accidents are often seen as primarily a matter of fate. This outlook is reflected in the very language we use to describe accidents. We talk about 'accidents waiting to happen', 'being in the wrong place at the wrong time', or our 'number' coming up. However, the striking regularity in accident patterns seen year after year shows that accidents are not determined by the chance fall of the dice. On the contrary, for accident patterns to replicate themselves in the same way year after year, there must be constant factors at work. It follows that if these factors could be identified we might have a starting point both for understanding what underlies accidents in the first place and for developing countermeasures aimed at preventing them. For this reason, the analysis of accident patterns is a major preoccupation in the field of accident epidemiology.

This chapter will review some of the major trends in accident patterns, especially pedestrian accidents, as they relate to children. We shall consider what they can tell us about the causes of such accidents; then move on to discuss what might be done to prevent them, focusing especially on what education might have to offer the child. Chapter 7 examines the effectiveness of current educational provision and how this might be improved. We shall pay particular attention to recent research suggesting that some fundamental changes are needed in how to approach this problem if children are to be given a better chance of survival on the roads.

ACCIDENTS IN PERSPECTIVE

Until comparatively recently, disease and infection were the major sources of morbidity and mortality in children. Indeed, throughout the early part of this century, parents would routinely wait in trepidation for the next outbreak of whooping cough, scarlet fever, tuberculosis or measles, knowing all too well what the consequences might be. Advances in medical science and primary health care have largely removed these terrors from late twentieth-century Europe, as is clearly illustrated in Figure 6.1. This shows the death rate per million children throughout the course of the twentieth century for some of the most life-threatening of childhood diseases. Notwithstanding the high mortality rates associated with these diseases in the early part of the century, it can be seen that most have been virtually eliminated from present-day Britain. The same cannot be said of accidents. Even by comparison to the cancers or congenital conditions which are much more difficult to control, accidents do not fare well. The result is that accidents now account for a far higher proportion of the deaths, injuries and long-term handicap in children than any of the traditional killer diseases of childhood, making them 'whether measured in terms of mortality or morbidity . . . the most important problem of child health today' (Jackson, 1978).

THE THREAT FROM ROAD ACCIDENTS

If accidents in general pose such a threat to children, how do road accidents fare by comparison? This question was addressed in a major World Health Organisation report in the 1980s which showed that, in Europe, between a third and a half of all accidental deaths to children occurred on the road (Deschamps, 1981). More recent figures in the UK are consistent with this trend. For example, in 1987 road deaths accounted for about two-thirds of all accidental deaths in children between the ages of 5 and 14 (O'Donoghue, 1988). In fact, road accidents are the leading cause of death for children under 15 years of age in most industrialised countries (Malek et al., 1990). Nor does the trend diminish as children get older: indeed, road accidents account for a *higher* proportion of deaths among 15–24 year-olds than in children, and remain the leading cause of death in adults under 35. However, a change takes place in the *type* of road accident that predominates in these older groups. Thus, whilst 15–24

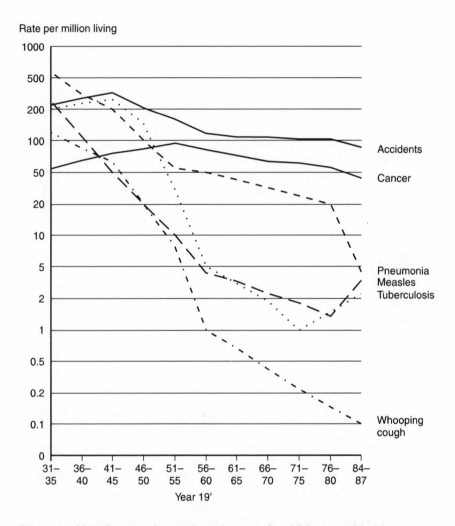

Rate per million living

Figure 6.1 Mortality rates from selected causes for children aged 1–14, England and Wales 1931–87 (rates per million population)

Source: OPCS. Deaths by cause. Quarterly Monitors DH2 88/3, 1988; Child Accident Prevention Trust, 1989

year-olds have more road accidents than children, these are predominantly accidents in which the victim was either the driver or a passenger in a vehicle. Most child victims, on the other hand, are pedestrians. This trend holds even though children spend much less time out and about on the streets than adults.

Assessing pedestrian vulnerability

In 1990, there were over 340,000 casualties on British roads, of whom more than 60,000 were pedestrians. This represents 18 per cent of all road casualties and 33 per cent of road deaths. This discrepancy follows from the fact that pedestrians are much less likely to survive an accident than the occupants of a vehicle, due to their relative lack of protection. Even so, the figures substantially *underestimate* pedestrians' vulnerability because they do not take the *exposure* of different categories of road user into account. Exposure is a complex concept but refers essentially to the fact that different categories of road user are not equally exposed to traffic: it follows that they are not equally exposed to risk. To understand this point, consider two neighbours with different appetites for seeing the world. The first stays at home and seldom goes out. The other is out and about all the time. Because he spends so much more time interacting with traffic, the second neighbour obviously has many more 'opportunities' to get knocked down than the first. In other words, he is more at risk. Therefore, the vulnerability of the two neighbours cannot be assessed just by counting the number of accidents they have had over a given period of time: we have to take into account the accompanying difference in exposure to traffic.

The same reasoning applies to different *groups* of road user. For example, if it turned out that, over a given time period, a group of 1,000 pedestrians had exactly the same number of accidents as a group of 1,000 drivers, we might be inclined to say that the risk of becoming a victim is equal in the two cases. But if we discovered that pedestrians are, in fact, much less exposed to traffic than drivers, the conclusion would not be true. In this case, the pedestrians would be more vulnerable. Indeed, one group of road users might actually have *fewer* accidents than another but, when exposure is taken into account, turn out to be more vulnerable. This is, in fact, true of cyclists in the UK, who have many fewer accidents than car drivers in absolute terms but who emerge as extremely vulnerable when their modest exposure to risk is taken into account (Department of Transport, 1993). In trying to determine who is most vulnerable on the road, then, we have to do much more than count the number of accidents: we must have a corresponding measure of exposure.

Measuring exposure to risk

Devising a measure to assess relative risk is no easy matter and satisfactory data are currently not available for all groups. The largest study that has attempted to collect such data is the UK Office of Population Censuses and Surveys, whose major analysis of pedestrian activity carried out in the late 1970s was undertaken specifically to derive exposure measures (Todd and Walker, 1980). The study used three measures to assess exposure: distance travelled per unit of time; number of roads crossed per unit of time; and amount of time spent walking over a given period. From these, three corresponding risk measures were derived: risk per road crossing; risk per kilometre walked; and risk per hour spent on foot. This is certainly an improvement on the more usual measure of accident rate per 100,000 population, but none of them offers a foolproof index of exposure. For example, two groups of pedestrians might cross the same number of roads over a given time span, but unless the roads contained similar volumes of traffic the comparison would not be very meaningful (Thomson, 1991). Comparisons between adults and children would be particularly susceptible to such distortions, because it is known that children cross a larger proportion of quiet streets than adults. The same bias would apply to the other two measures described above. Some authors have proposed 'number of encounters with a vehicle' as a more appropriate measure (e.g. Routledge et al., 1974a), but deriving this measure is rather difficult.

In any event, when an effort is made to obtain a realistic picture of pedestrian risk by taking exposure into account, the vulnerability of pedestrians emerges as far higher than the actual number of accidents would suggest. The Department of Transport estimates that the risk of becoming a pedestrian casualty is no less than *15 times higher* than when travelling by car. Only motor cycling turns out to be a more dangerous form of transport when calculated in this way (O'Donoghue, 1988). This is a disturbing finding in itself; but the estimate applies only to *adult* pedestrians, because the Todd and Walker study did not measure children's traffic exposure (studies are currently under way with the aim of producing a more comprehensive picture of the risk to different groups of pedestrian, including children). As we shall see below, smaller-scale studies aimed at estimating child pedestrian risk produce estimates of truly epidemic proportions.

TRENDS IN CHILD PEDESTRIAN ACCIDENTS

Pedestrian accident patterns vary markedly as a function of age. For example, 90 per cent of the injuries and over half the fatalities involving children under the age of five occur in the home (Kravitz, 1973). Obviously, this reflects the fact that very young children spend little time outside the home and their exposure to traffic is therefore low. Once children reach school age, however, the picture changes dramatically, with pedestrian casualties increasing by around 300 per cent (Thomson, 1989). Moreover, the trend continues to grow for several years so that, in most countries, children in the age range 5–9 years suffer approximately four times as many accidents as adults.

Historically, 5–9 year-olds have suffered the highest casualty rate of all age groups but, more recently, a worrying trend has developed among 10–14 year-olds who have traditionally suffered a slightly lower casualty rate. Recently, this group's accident rate has been increasing relative to most others, whose rates have either decreased or remained stable. In fact, since 1985 accident rates in 10–14 year-olds actually overtook 5–9 year-olds for the first time, a trend that has been maintained over the subsequent decade (Department of Transport, 1993). The trend has obvious implications for the sort of road safety education these older children might need and requires careful monitoring. It also has implications for the adequacy of the training they received at a younger age, and the extent to which this helped them prepare for the traffic situations they are expected to cope with once they become 10–14 year-olds. We return to this point in the next chapter.

A further prominent feature of child pedestrian accidents is the marked gender difference that is found. The effect is not specific to any one country but has been reliably replicated in countries across the globe. The difference is particularly marked in the vulnerable 5–9 year age group, with boys suffering twice as many accidents as girls. However, a similar bias is found in all age groups except the over 70s, with males having roughly 40 per cent more accidents than females. The bias is found even among 0–4 year-olds. Although this gender effect is very powerful, it has proved extremely elusive and no straightforward reasons can be given to explain it. Part of the explanation may lie in exposure differences between boys and girls but this cannot be a complete answer as the effect persists in cases where exposure is known to be about equal (Routledge *et al.*, 1974a). Many authors refer to differences in road behaviour and more risk-taking by boys but, again, the data presented never look convincing as an overall explanation. In spite of the magnitude of this sex difference, we honestly cannot say with confidence what factors are primarily responsible for it. It remains one of the most interesting challenges to road safety research at the present time (for reviews of this topic, see Foot, 1985, and Thomson, 1991).

Finally, we should not let this concern with children's vulnerability obscure the fact that one other group is also disproportionately threatened by the road environment. This group is the elderly, especially those over the age of 75. The elderly are vulnerable not so much because they have an especially high overall accident rate (at least relative to children) but because the accidents they do suffer have much more serious consequences. In fact, fatalities among the elderly account for 25 per cent of all pedestrian fatalities. This, of course, reflects the frailty of older people and their limited ability to recover from any injuries they sustain.

However unwelcome these figures might be, it must again be realised that they almost certainly *underestimate* the risk faced by children on the road. Although national surveys have not yet produced data on the exposure of children to traffic, studies conducted on a smaller scale have provided evidence of marked differences between adults and children (as well as between older and younger children). The reason lies in the fact that, over comparable time periods, children cross *fewer roads* than adults; the roads they do cross are *less busy*; and they generally spend *less time* in traffic (Routledge *et al.*, 1974a, 1974b; van der Molen, 1981b). There is therefore a lower probability (in terms of exposure) of children having an accident in the first place. Any assessment of the risk to child pedestrians must take this into account.

The picture that emerges when accident data are supplemented by exposure data in this way is that the former grossly underestimate the scale of the problem. For example, Routledge *et al.*'s estimates suggest that children between the ages of 5 and 7 are as much as *40 times* as vulnerable as adults in the age range 20–50. Yet adult pedestrians are themselves 15 times more likely to become casualties than are the occupants of vehicles. Another important finding is that, when exposure is taken into account, major roads emerge as more dangerous to young children than minor ones. By contrast, adults are no more vulnerable on one than on the other. This is consistent with the idea that adults are skilled in dealing with the road (hence busy roads are not particularly dangerous for them). By contrast, children are more vulnerable on such roads because they do not yet have the skills to deal with them. This emphasises their lack of experience and highlights the importance of education.

SOCIAL CLASS

Along with age and sex, social class is the other major factor that emerges from the accident statistics, with children from lower socio-economic groups having a disproportionately large number of accidents of all types (Langley, 1984). Indeed, accidents seem to produce a steeper social class gradient than any other cause of death (Townsend and Davidson, 1988). Preston (1972) found that road accidents correlated highly with indices of crowding and social class, a finding confirmed by Read *et al.* (1963), who found accidents to be commoner in areas of dense, multi-dwelling housing associated with inner city areas. The same finding has been obtained more recently in a large study by Lawson (1990), who also found greater vulnerability in certain ethnic groups. However, the latter finding is probably an artefact of the fact that so many ethnic groups live in vulnerable inner city areas in the first place. Vulnerable communites are not restricted to the inner city, however: in urban Scotland, many high accident, low SES areas are concentrated in the large peripheral housing schemes developed during the post-war period as means of alleviating slum conditions. Such areas often generate very high child accident rates (Ampofo-Boateng, 1987; Thomson, 1993).

However, whilst the relationship between accident rates and social class is fairly clear, it is much less obvious how the relationship should be accounted for. Exposure differences seem likely to partially explain the effects. For example, in inner-city areas traffic volumes are high, thereby predisposing children to risk. Similarly, lack of gardens or protected playing spaces are likely to drive children on to the streets where their exposure would again be increased. However, it is sometimes suggested that there may also be behavioural differences between children from different social class backgrounds that interact with exposure in determining vulnerability. Factors such as family size, unemployment, divorce or marital discord, physical or mental illness in the family, and supposedly poor or ineffectual parental child-rearing practices have all been proposed as relevant factors that are more prevalent in disadvantaged social groups (see Thomson, 1991, for a review). Obviously, if such factors affected parental supervision and the like, this might increase children's vulnerability. However, very little is known about the extent to which these factors do, in fact, affect parental supervision and we are really not in a position to disentangle them from the fact that low SES children are far more likely to live in an intrinsically more dangerous environment than the middle classes. Nevertheless, the fact that accidents can be localised to particular areas should at the very least help identify those children most in need of support, whether through measures aimed at reducing traffic speed and the volume of traffic in an area; the creation of parks, recreational areas and so on; or increased educational provision, showing children (and their parents) how better to cope with traffic situations.

WHEN DO ACCIDENTS HAPPEN?

Pedestrian accidents tend to be higher during the final quarter of the year, i.e. during October, November and December, though the effect is not marked. There are somewhat fewer accidents during January and February, presumably because the weather reduces the amount of time people spend out of doors. Fewer accidents take place on Sundays than other days of the week, again reflecting reduced traffic activity on that day.

Pedestrians are somewhat more likely to get knocked down during the hours of darkness than at other times. For children, however, the most dangerous time to be out on foot is between 8 and 9 o'clock in the morning and between 3 and 6 o'clock in the afternoon. These times obviously coincide with the morning and evening rush hours and with the journey to and from school. In fact, 20 per cent of accidents among 5–9 year-olds take place on school journeys, a figure that rises to no less than

40 per cent in the case of 10–14 year-olds. At weekends, these morning and evening peaks disappear and are replaced by a higher accident rate during the main part of the day (when on schooldays children would be in class and therefore not exposed to risk). The school journey is thus a very vulnerable period for schoolchildren of all ages. If road safety were to concentrate on investigating the circumstances surrounding accidents on such journeys and perhaps help children find the safest possible routes for their own particular journey to school, this might have substantial benefits.

WHERE DO ACCIDENTS TAKE PLACE?

As you would expect, 95 per cent of accidents occur in built-up areas – though a disproportionately large number of fatalities occur in non-built-up areas. This presumably reflects the higher speeds at which vehicles travel on such roads. Although busy roads are obviously dangerous, it is surprising how many accidents take place on quiet roads where traffic volumes are relatively low. In adults, 50 per cent of accidents occur on such minor roads: in children under 9 years of age the proportion rises to 80 per cent. This difference between adults and children reflects exposure differences but it is a salutary lesson to realise how dangerous quiet roads are, even for adults. In children, as many as 60 per cent of accidents occur within a quarter mile of the child's home and a large proportion actually take place in the street where the child lives (Grayson, 1975; Chapman et al., 1982).

One problem in trying to reduce such accidents is that the volume of traffic in such areas is generally too low for the local authorities to feel justified in installing crossing facilities; although there has developed in recent years a very welcome trend towards the introduction of (admittedly low-cost) measures aimed at reducing traffic speed. The result is that anyone crossing such roads is forced to rely on his or her own skill in doing so. Since pedestrian skills are poorly developed in young children, they may even be more vulnerable on minor roads than on some busier ones where crossing facilities do exist. Yet quiet suburban roads are precisely the ones that parents are most likely to think their children can tackle alone. The trouble is that such roads do not *look* dangerous. Nevertheless, children end up with four times the adult accident rate by trying to cross such roads. The fact is, there is no such thing as a 'safe street' for young, inexperienced pedestrians. This emphasises just how vulnerable children are and how important it is to devise effective educational interventions for them.

WHY DO CHILDREN HAVE ACCIDENTS?

The evidence that emerges from an analysis of the accident data is that children are vulnerable to injury wherever and whenever they interact with traffic. The vulnerability is not reserved for busy roads or other exceptionally dangerous situations. In fact, the majority of accidents take place on relatively quiet residential streets. It is hard to avoid the conclusion that the child's inexperience must be a factor.

It is generally agreed that children do not begin to approach adult levels of pedestrian skill until around 11 years of age (Thomson, 1991). Even then, they do not appear to deploy these skills very effectively, as the continuing high accident rate among 10–14 year-olds makes clear. However, it is younger children, and especially those under 9 years of age, who make the weakest traffic judgements and are therefore least well equipped to deal with the hazards of the road. These trends are reflected in long-standing government advice that children should not be exposed to traffic on their own until they are at least 10 years of age. In practice, very few people follow this advice in a rigorous way and it seems likely that most children are permitted at least a degree of traffic experience well before this. In addition, it is a matter of common observation that many children are permitted access to traffic at an astonishingly early age. It would seem that parents' perceptions of their children's skill are not entirely in tune with those of the government. We return to this in the next chapter.

It is all very well to say that young children lack the experience to cope with traffic, but this is not very helpful in deciding what can be done about it. Exactly which aspects of experience is it that children lack? Could children be given the necessary experience through educational intervention? Or are children intrinsically limited in the skills they can acquire until a certain age has been reached? These questions have long preoccupied researchers in road safety and continue to be a major source of controversy at the present time. It is to these issues that we now turn.

TRADITIONAL APPROACHES TO ROAD SAFETY EDUCATION

Although the whole road safety field is currently engaged in very active re-examination of its aims and activities (see the next chapter), it is still the case that most road safety education takes place in the classroom with the aim of increasing children's *knowledge* about traffic and their *attitudes* towards safety. The instruction is almost entirely verbal: that is, children learn by being *told* about traffic rather than by actually *doing* anything. The idea is that, by building up a knowledge base and set of appropriate attitudes towards their own safety, children will be able to generalise what they have learned in class to the concrete traffic situations that will confront them on the street.

Many resources have been developed in an effort to do this. Traditionally, road safety was based around occasional visits from police or road safety training officers, with the school being urged to follow up on these visits with additional work and activities. A wide range of printed materials have been developed for this purpose, together with a certain number of films, videos, slide presentations and similar resources. Occasionally, radio or television productions for schools broadcasting have also been produced. Relatively few practical activities or exercises have been devised in which children would take a more participative role, although simple simulations of a road or zebra crossing might be set up in the school gym or playground. There are certainly none of the more sophisticated traffic parks and gardens that have been developed as resources in other European countries. However, in recent years a number of 'traffic trails' and similar schemes have been developed in which children receive some road safety education in the real road environment whilst out on a specially designed trail with their teachers (e.g. Davies *et al.*, 1993). Such approaches using real roads as the context for training are much to be welcomed. It remains to be seen how widespread their use will become or how much training children will actually receive in this way.

The Green Cross Code

By far the most important aid to road safety education developed in the UK is the Green Cross Code, a short set of simple verbal rules aimed at providing children with a general purpose strategy for crossing the road. It was introduced in the early 1970s as a replacement for the much older Kerb Drill (introduced in 1942), which was by then regarded as old-fashioned and rather militaristic in tone (it contained commands such as 'Halt!' and 'Quick March!'). It was also felt that children could often recite the drill correctly but apply it in a rather 'blind', uncomprehending fashion at the roadside. The tendency of young children to apply rules rigidly, almost as if they were a talisman to ward off danger, is an important feature of children's behaviour. The Kerb Drill was eventually replaced by the more flexible Green Cross Code, which has occupied a central place in UK road safety education ever since. The basic precepts of the Code are:

First find a safe place to cross, then stop.
Stand on the pavement near the kerb.
Look all round for traffic and listen.
If traffic is coming, let it pass, look all round again.
When there is no traffic near, walk straight across the road.
Keep looking and listening for traffic while you cross.

The Code was tested on a sample of 7 and 8 year-old children to see whether they could read it satisfactorily and could go through the steps described in an adequate manner (Sargent and Sheppard, 1974). The conclusion was that children of this age would be able to read and follow the instructions without too much difficulty, although it was likely that the injunction to find a safe place would probably prove too difficult for them. This turns out to be of great significance, as we shall see. Later studies conducted on 5 and 6 year-olds suggested that this age group was much less likely to be able to learn the Code and the authors suggested that a different approach might be required with this age group (Fisk and Cliff, 1975). In due course, a simpler version was produced (Stop, Look, Listen, Think) which is now used as an introduction to road safety for younger children.

HOW EFFECTIVE IS TRADITIONAL ROAD SAFETY EDUCATION?

The question that arises is, how effective are these methods in teaching children about traffic and the traffic environment? Unfortunately, the answer is not encouraging. It is certainly undeniable that approaches aimed at knowledge acquisition do increase children's knowledge about traffic. Unfortunately, there is no evidence that this knowledge generalises to their behaviour at the roadside. Thus, while the children may give more informed answers when questioned in the classroom, there is no evidence that they do anything differently when they are out on the street. Even when researchers have carried out behavioural (as opposed to verbal) tests immediately after the class, there is scant evidence that the children behave differently. Numerous studies have assessed road safety education in this way and the conclusion really seems indisputable: if the aim of road safety education is to get children to behave in a safer and more skilful way at the roadside, then purely knowledge-based approaches do not work (for extensive reviews on this issue, see Rothengatter, 1981; Thomson, 1991).

In spite of the fact that road accidents constitute one of the gravest threats to children in the modern world, it seems that efforts at educating children to cope more successfully with traffic have led to limited success. Some authorities have suggested that the reduction in accidents as a result of education may be as low as 10 per cent (Howarth and Repetto-Wright, 1978): others have suggested that there may simply be a limit to what can be achieved with children until they reach a certain age, usually taken to be around 10 years (Sandels, 1975). Whatever the truth of this, a sense of malaise has certainly been detectable in the field for some time and there has developed a growing tendency to focus on alternative means of dealing with the problem, such as making the traffic environment safer in the first place.

This latter trend is a very welcome one. There is no doubt that the layout of road networks, including those in many residential districts, has made them intrinsically more dangerous than need be and it is right that efforts should be made to rectify this. In some countries such as the Netherlands, major urban planning initiatives have been introduced together with substantial traffic legislation in order to do this. Among the most important has been the creation of special residential areas (*woonerven*), where pedestrians have legal priority over traffic at all times. These 'safe havens' enjoy much lower accident rates than comparable areas in the UK. Unfortunately, the creation of such districts is expensive and carries major legislative implications. Little effort has been made to follow the Dutch example in this country.

In the UK, the approach has been towards the introduction of low-cost measures, mainly aimed at reducing vehicle speeds. This has been accomplished through the introduction of road bumps, chicanes, speed tables and similar devices aimed at forcing drivers to reduce speed in areas where they might otherwise drive faster. This aim is desirable because lower speeds should result in fewer pedestrian accidents in all age groups. In addition, where an accident does occur, the effects should be less severe. It therefore seems likely that these measures will become more widespread – a wholly desirable development.

On the negative side, it has to be said that such measures are invariably introduced sparingly, mainly to roads where there is clear evidence of a problem. There appears to be no likelihood of their being implemented on a wide scale and no likelihood whatever that whole residential districts will be turned into *woonerven*. Thus, the need for education is a continuing one. It must also be remembered that the vast majority of child pedestrian accidents occur on roads with relatively low volumes of traffic and where vehicle speeds are also relatively low in any case: certainly too low for local authorities to consider installing crossing facilities. The fact is, it is hard to imagine a traffic environment where there would be no need for pedestrian skills. So long as there are roads at all, children will have to learn how to use them

CAN ROAD SAFETY SKILLS BE TAUGHT?

We have seen that, in general, most of the approaches to road safety education attempted to date have met with limited success. The question arises as to why this should be. Have we simply been teaching the wrong things? Or can road safety not really be taught effectively to children until they have reached some prior stage of development? Is it reasonable to expect young children to acquire and demonstrate the abilities needed to interact with traffic? We have seen that children have difficulty even in learning the Green Cross Code until they are 7 or 8 years of age. Does this represent a lower limit on the age at which serious road safety education should begin? And given that children do not normally approach adult levels of performance until around 11–12 years of age, is it actually possible to improve significantly the performance of younger children through education?

The answer that has generally been given to these questions is 'no'. At best, it has been argued that there is a clear limit to what younger children can learn until an appropriate stage of psychological development has been reached. This point of view was first stated by Sandels (1975) on the basis of her extensive pioneering research into child pedestrian behaviour in Sweden. Sandels' work included extensive observational studies of children interacting with traffic, both when at play in the street and when engaged in more purposeful activities like going to the shops. She also conducted a range of laboratory-based experiments into the perceptual and cognitive abilities that seemed important to traffic behaviour, such as sound localisation (although these were not of a technically high order) and she conducted extensive interviews with both children and their parents. On the basis of this work, Sandels came to the now famous conclusion that 'it is not possible to adapt fully young children (under 10 years) to the traffic environment. They are biologically incapable of managing its many demands' (Sandels, 1975). Her recommendation was that efforts should be aimed primarily at separating children from traffic altogether. Other leading researchers such as Vinjé (1981) have also stressed children's limitations, though Vinjé expressed a good deal more optimism as to what might be achieved through education and training. Indeed, her paper heralded an extensive educational research programme in the Netherlands that has guided traffic education for Dutch children ever since (van der Molen, 1989). Nevertheless, Vinjé's emphasis was on adapting pedestrian strategies to the more limited skills that could be assumed in young children. There was no consideration that the skills themselves could be taught.

Characteristics of the pre-operational child

This outlook stems directly from a common interpretation of Jean Piaget's enormously influential theory of development (e.g. Piaget, 1955). According to this theory, development proceeds by way of four main stages: the sensori-motor stage (0–2 years), the pre-operational stage (2–7 years), the concrete operational stage (7–11 years) and the formal operational stage (11 years upwards). From the road safety point of view, the characteristics of pre-operational thinking are particularly pertinent because certain mental operations that would appear to be necessary in making accurate pedestrian judgements have not yet developed at this stage. In particular, pre-operational children have difficulty with any task in which two or more variables have to be combined – or, indeed, appreciating that more than one variable is at work at all.

A particularly pertinent example in the context of road safety is the 'two trains task' in which the child must say which of two trains will arrive at a destination first (Piaget, 1969). Since the trains start from different points and travel at different speeds, the child must grasp the relationship between speed and distance in order to come up with the correct answer. According to Piaget, children are unable to differentiate time and space until the age of 8–9 years and so make many errors on this and similar tasks. In general, younger children tend to fixate on a single cue and ignore the others. In the two trains task, distance usually proves more salient than velocity and the children argue that the train which is *closer* to the destination will arrive first – even if the other train is travelling faster. As a result, children make many incorrect time-to-arrival judgements. Since such time-to-arrival judgements are obviously required at the roadside, the implication of Piaget's findings for road safety is obvious.

A further characteristic of pre-operational thinking with implications for road safety is that children at this stage often have difficulty in adopting the perspective of another person, both literally and metaphorically. Just as pre-operational children fixate on single variables in the two trains task, so they fixate on their own point of view when looking at a scene and fail to realise that other views are possible. Typically, the children will attribute to other observers the same view of the object or scene that they themselves enjoy (Piaget and Inhelder, 1956). It has been suggested that this effect, known as *egocentricity*, may underlie the tendency of children to think that if they can see the driver of an approaching vehicle, then the driver can also see them. Such errors would be particularly dangerous when the child is actually hidden from the driver's view, as is often the case when crossing near parked cars or other obstructions (Ampofo-Boateng and Thomson, 1991).

Such findings have obvious implications for road safety education because they point to limitations in the judgements that can be expected of children under 8 or 9 years of age. The critical issue is whether children's ability to solve such problems can be accelerated. Piaget argued that the four developmental stages must be passed through in a fixed order (i.e. the child cannot 'jump' a stage) and he specified ages by which he expected most children would attain each stage, given the experience and education typically enjoyed by children in Western societies. A common interpretation of Piaget in the 1960s and early 1970s, particularly in educational circles, was that the theory is fundamentally maturational in character and that the stages pose *biological limitations* on the rate of development. From this comes the idea, very common among educationalists, that children can only be taught certain things 'when they are ready'. If true, this would mean that little, if any, acceleration of such basic skills could be expected as a result of education or training. The appropriate action would be simply to protect children from traffic 'until childhood has matured out of them' (Sandels, 1975). In general, this is held to occur around 9 years of age.

PROMOTING DEVELOPMENT IN YOUNG CHILDREN: CAN IT BE DONE?

This point of view is a very pessimistic one for road safety education, because it implies that little can be done at an educational level. In turn, this would shift the emphasis away from education altogether towards engineering and urban planning measures aimed at creating an intrinsically safer environment. The relative lack of impact made by traditional road safety education has certainly fuelled this view. However, such a view is both too optimistic about the benefits of engineering and too pessimistic about the limitations of education. Several issues lead to this conclusion and should encourage us to be more optimistic about what education can achieve. First of all, contemporary developmental psychologists are far less convinced about the inflexibility of the Piagetian stages than some earlier writers appear to have been. Indeed, a large body of research since the mid-1970s has comprehensively demonstrated that children frequently can learn to solve problems ahead of the supposedly 'correct' developmental stage, and sometimes far in advance of it. Whether or not this happens depends on numerous factors associated, for example, with the language and methodology used and the precise way in which the task is set up (for a review, see Donaldson, 1978). A good deal of current developmental psychology is concerned with these processes (e.g. Boden, 1994). The situation thus seems far from as inflexible as has often been assumed. The broad sweep of contemporary psychological research is certainly not consistent with the simplistic view that development is constrained to follow a fixed, age-determined path and is not amenable to intervention through education.

In addition, there has recently been an upsurge of interest in empirical investigations aimed at accelerating development, and some of this research has been conducted in the context of road safety. For example, roadside training programmes aimed at improving visual timing skills have been undertaken with children as young as 5 years of age with extremely encouraging results (e.g. Lee, Young and McLaughlin, 1984; Young and Lee, 1987; van Schagen, 1988; Demetre et al., 1992, 1993). Similarly, the effectiveness of training in improving the ability of 5 year-olds to find safe places to cross the road has been demonstrated in recent studies by Thomson (1993); Thomson et al. (1993); Tucker (1993); and Ampofo-Boateng et al. (1993). Even studies aimed at reducing children's

vulnerability to distraction and impulsive behaviour have been undertaken with encouraging results (Limbourg and Gerber, 1978). Thus, there
are both theoretical and empirical reasons for questioning whether
children are as limited in what they can learn as has been supposed.
Perhaps road safety education has failed because children are not being
taught what they really need to know. In addition, it is possible that the
teaching methods may not be appropriate. These possibilities are explored
in the next chapter.

SUMMARY

To place child pedestrian accidents in perspective, there is no doubt that
they pose one of the foremost threats to the health and well-being of
children in the modern world. Yet it is astonishing how lightly this
situation is accepted. Most parents seem only dimly aware of the extent
and the potency of the threat and are typically far more worried by
situations which are, in fact, far less threatening. For example, although
parents now allow their children much less freedom to go out than they
did some twenty years ago (Hillman *et al.*, 1990), this is far more likely to
be conditioned by fears of abduction by strangers or attack from a
Rottweiler than by recognition of the far more real threats posed by
traffic. The former threats, serious as they may be, are insignificant by
comparison. Perhaps the answer is that child pedestrian accidents ac-
cumulate insidiously, building up in ones and twos across the country
rather than in sensational form. Certainly, they lack the drama of airline
crashes, motorway pile-ups and the like. Since such highly visible events
inevitably attract a great deal of media attention, it is perhaps not surprising that the public's perception largely reflects the scale and frequency of
such reports. Ironically, it may be the very fact that pedestrian accidents
are commonplace that leads to their passing unremarked.

Although educational countermeasures have been in use for a
considerable time, it is unclear just how effective these have been in
combating accidents. Increasing children's traffic knowledge and attempting to instil positive attitudes towards safety may sound like a
reasonable means of changing the way children behave in traffic but it is
hard to find much evidence that it is. It has been suggested that this may
reflect limitations posed by the natural process of psychological development and that there may be a limit to what realistically can be achieved
through education. This outlook may be too pessimistic, however. Are
children really so limited in what they can learn? Or is it possible that
road safety education has not been teaching the right things in the right
way? If we took a different approach could things be different? It is to
these questions that we now turn.

REFERENCES

Ampofo-Boateng, K. (1987) 'Children's perception of safety and danger on the road', unpublished Ph.D. dissertation, University of Strathclyde.

Ampofo-Boateng, K. and Thomson, J. A. (1991) 'Children's perception of safety and danger on the road', *British Journal of Psychology* 82: 487–505.

Ampofo-Boateng, K., Thomson, J. A., Grieve, R., Pitcairn, T., Lee, D. N. and Demetre, J. D. (1993) 'A developmental and training study of children's ability to find safe routes to cross the road', *British Journal of Developmental Psychology* 11: 31–45.

Boden, M. A. (1994) *Piaget*, London: Fontana.

Chapman, A. J., Wade, F. M. and Foot, H. C. (eds) (1982) *Pedestrian Accidents*, Chichester: Wiley.

Davies, J., Guy, J. and Murray, G. (1993) 'You decide to stay alive: a child pedestrian project, years 1–3', Transport Research Laboratory Report PR/SRC/15/9, Crowthorne: TRL.

Demetre, J. D., Lee, D. N., Pitcairn, T. K., Grieve, R., Thomson, J. A. and Ampofo-Boateng, K. (1992) 'Errors in young children's decisions about traffic gaps: experiments with roadside simulations', *British Journal of Psychology* 83: 189–202.

Demetre, J. D., Lee, D. N., Grieve, R., Pitcairn, T. K., Ampofo-Boateng, K. and Thomson, J. A. (1993) 'Young children's learning on road-crossing simulations', *British Journal of Educational Psychology* 63: 348–58.

Department of Transport (1993) *Road Accidents Great Britain 1992: The Casualty Report*, London: HMSO.

Deschamps, J. P. (1981) *Prevention of Traffic Accidents in Childhood*, Copenhagen: World Health Organisation.

Donaldson, M. (1978) *Children's Minds*, Glasgow: Fontana.

Fisk, A. and Cliff, H. (1975) 'The effects of teaching the Green Cross Code to young children', Department of the Environment Report 168UC, Crowthorne: TRL.

Foot, H. C. (1985) 'Boys will be boys?', *Safety Education* 1: 1–6.

Grayson, G. B. (1975) 'The Hampshire child pedestrian accident study', Department of the Environment Report 670, Crowthorne: TRRL.

Hillman, M., Adams, J. and Whitelegg, J. (1990) *One False Move . . . A Study of Children's Independent Mobility*, London: Institute for Policy Studies.

Howarth, C. I. and Repetto-Wright, R. (1978) 'Measurement of risk and the attribution of responsibility for child pedestrian accidents', *Safety Education* 144: 10–13.

Jackson, R. H. (1978) *Children, the Environment and Accidents*, London: Pitman Medical.

Kravitz, A. (1973) 'Accident prevention research', *Paediatric Annals* 2: 47–53.

Langley, J. (1984) 'Injury control – psychosocial considerations', *Journal of Child Psychology and Psychiatry* 25: 349–56.

Lawson, S. D. (1990) *Accidents to Young Pedestrians: Distributions, Circumstances, Consequences and Scope for Countermeasures*, Basingstoke: AA Foundation for Road Safety Research.

Lee, D. N., Young, D. S. and McLaughlin, C. M. (1984) 'A roadside simulation of road crossing for young children', *Ergonomics* 17: 319–30.

Limbourg, M. and Gerber, D. (1978) 'A parent training program for the road safety education of preschool children', *Accident Analysis and Prevention* 13: 255–67.

Malek, M., Guyer, B. and Lescohier, I. (1990) 'The epidemiology and prevention of child pedestrian injury', *Accident Analysis and Prevention* 22: 301–13.

Molen, H. H. van der (1981a) 'Blueprint of an analysis of the pedestrian task-1: method of analysis', *Accident Analysis and Prevention* 13: 175–91.

—— (1981b) 'Child pedestrian's exposure, accidents and behaviour', *Accident Analysis and Prevention* 13: 193–224.

—— (1989) 'World pedestrian training: experience and possibilities for world wide application', *World Safety Journal* 111: 23–25.

O'Donoghue, J. (1988) 'Pedestrian accidents', in *Road Accidents Great Britain: The Casualty Report 1987*, London: HMSO.

Piaget, J. (1955) 'Les stades du développement intellectuel de l'enfant et de l'adolescent', in P. Osterrieth (ed.) *Le Problème des Stades en Psychologie de L'Enfant*, Paris: Presses Universitaires de France.

—— (1969) *The Child's Conception of Time*, London: Routledge and Kegan Paul.

Piaget, J. and Inhelder, B. (1956) *The Child's Conception of Space*, London: Routledge and Kegan Paul.

Preston, B. (1972) 'Statistical analysis of child pedestrian accidents in Manchester and Salford', *Accident Analysis and Prevention* 4: 323–32.

Read, J. H., Bradley, E. J., Morrison, J. D., Lewell, D. and Clarke, D. A. (1963) 'The epidemiology and prevention of traffic accidents involving young children', *Canadian Medical Association Journal* 989: 687–701.

Rothengatter, J. A. (1981) *Traffic Safety Education for Young Children*, Lisse: Swets and Reitlinger.

Routledge, D. A., Repetto-Wright, R. and Howarth, C. I. (1974a) 'The exposure of young children to accident risk as pedestrians', *Ergonomics* 17: 457–80.

—— (1974b) 'A comparison of interviews and observations to obtain measures of children's exposure to risk as pedestrians', *Ergonomics* 17: 623–38.

Sandels, S. (1975) *Children in Traffic*, London: Elek.

Sargent, K. J. and Sheppard, D. (1974) 'The development of the Green Cross Code', Department of the Environment Report LR605, Crowthorne: TRRL.

Schagen, van I. (1988) 'Training children to make safe crossing decisions', in J. A. Rothengatter and R. A. de Bruin (eds) *Road User Behaviour:Theory and Practice*, Assen: Van Gorum.

Thomson, J. A. (1989) 'Safe to school: improving road safety education', *Scottish Council for Research in Education Newsletter*, 44: 4–5.

—— (1991) *The Facts about Child Pedestrian Accidents*, London: Cassell.

—— (1993) 'A community approach to the teaching of pedestrian skills in young children', paper presented at 'Recent Developments and Research in Road Safety', University of Salford.

Thomson, J. A., Ampofo-Boateng, K., Pitcairn, T., Grieve, R., Lee, D. N. and Demetre, J. D. (1992) 'Behavioural group training of children to find safe routes to cross the road', *British Journal of Educational Psychology*, 62: 173–83.

Todd, J. E. and Walker, A. (1980) *People as Pedestrians*, London: HMSO.

Townsend, P. and Davidson, P. (1988) *The Black Report*, Harmondsworth: Penguin.

Tucker, S. (1993) 'A pedestrian training resource for children aged 5 to 8', Transport Research Laboratory Report PR/SRC/16/93, Crowthorne: TRL.

Vinjé, M. P. (1981) 'Children as pedestrians: abilities and limitations', *Accident Analysis and Prevention* 13: 225–40.

Young, D. S. and Lee, D. N. (1987) 'Training children in road crossing skills using a roadside simulation', *Accident Analysis and Prevention* 19: 327–41.

Chapter 7

Increasing traffic competence in young children

James A. Thomson

PROBLEMS OF RULE-BASED APPROACHES TO ROAD SAFETY EDUCATION

In the last chapter we saw that simply increasing children's knowledge about road safety does not seem to influence the way they *behave* when confronted with real traffic situations. Even approaches that do place more emphasis on behaviour, like the Green Cross Code, are taught verbally and the effectiveness of teaching is assessed by the extent to which children can recite it on demand. It is *assumed* that if children can do this, they will be able to turn what they recite into appropriate behaviour at the roadside.

Unfortunately, this assumption does not appear to be warranted. Even when children do attempt to put the Code into practice, they often do so in a rather rigid and inappropriate manner without properly understanding what it is they are meant to do. For example, when asked to 'look for cars' it is not uncommon to see children faithfully moving their heads from side to side but at such speed as to have no chance of seeing anything! Sometimes, the child appears to think that what they are being asked to do is simply to make head movements. This tendency to apply rules rigidly is common in younger children. The likelihood of their doing so increases when the rules are taught in an inappropriate context. Obviously, traffic rules learned verbally in the classroom fall into this category.

Consistent with this view is the finding that quite a lot of accidents happen to children who did, in fact, look for traffic but somehow *failed to see it* (e.g. Grayson, 1975a; MVA, 1989). This probably happens when children go through the motions without really understanding what the adult means by 'look'. What the child is, in fact, being asked to do is make a whole series of visual judgements: detecting whether vehicles are present in the first place; if they are, determining their distance; their velocity; their direction of travel; whether they are accelerating or decelerating; and so on. 'Looking' for traffic thus implies a wide range of judgements that are so self-evident to experienced pedestrians that they fail to make them explicit when talking to a child. Unfortunately, these nuances may entirely escape the novice pedestrian. It is therefore essential that road safety education should make as explicit as possible what the child is expected to do. Inexperienced children simply cannot be expected to make these links for themselves. Again, the more the teaching is divorced from the context in which the children will be expected to apply the rules, the lower the chances that they will make the links (Thomson, 1991). Classroom-based teaching, focusing on rules learned in the abstract, clearly runs this risk.

It cannot be assumed, then, that learning rules or increasing knowledge *per se* will lead to improved behaviour at the roadside. Nor should we be unduly surprised by this: as Lee *et al.* (1984) point out, no-one would expect to learn to drive just sitting at a desk! One reason why road safety education has not been particularly successful may be that it has not been teaching the right things in the right way. Rather than learning to give answers to questions about road safety, what children really need is *practical experience* of dealing with traffic situations (albeit in a safe and controlled manner). What kind of traffic situations should they be introduced to? What practical skills do pedestrians need in order to deal with them effectively? Such questions go to the heart of road safety education because, unless we can explicitly state what competences children need, we have no way of setting aims and objectives in order to achieve them.

WHAT SHOULD ROAD SAFETY EDUCATION TEACH?

The major shortcoming of most current road safety education is that it lacks a clear appreciation of the skills needed to deal with the traffic environment. As a result, it is unclear what should be taught. In fact, remarkably few educational countermeasures attempt to specify in any detail what their objectives are or indicate why these should be expected to make the child safer on the road (Rothengatter, 1981; Thomson *et al.*, 1994). There almost seems to be an assumption that if material deals with road safety at all, then it is bound to have a beneficial effect. Unfortunately, there is no justification for so optimistic a view.

A more scientific way of establishing objectives would be to analyse the *problems* posed by the traffic environment; the *strategies* by which an experienced pedestrian might solve such problems; and the underlying *skills* required in order for appropriate strategic behaviour to be possible. In many ways, this would seem to be an obvious starting point for the development of educational objectives. For example, if it could be shown that children lack the skills needed to tackle a particular road task, an appropriate educational objective might be to teach those skills. If children are unable to benefit from such training until a certain age has been reached, it might nevertheless be possible to teach a more limited strategy that would suit the skill level of younger children. In the extreme case, it might be necessary to recommend that the child should not tackle certain road tasks at all. However, all such advice and recommendations should be based on solid empirical evidence concerning the skills that children possess at different ages and on whether or not it is possible to accelerate acquisition of the skills through training.

What exactly does a skilled pedestrian need to be able to do in order to cope successfully with the road environment? After all, crossing the road seems a pretty straightforward affair to most people, and it might be asked what all the fuss is about. In fact, this common view is a severely misguided one. Road crossing involves a wide range of complex per-ceptual, cognitive and motor skills without which skilled pedestrian behaviour would be impossible. Adult pedestrians demonstrate con-siderable competence in applying these to the pedestrian task. Children, on the other hand, do not. Thus, a credible aim of road safety education might be to enhance these skills and show how they should be applied in different traffic contexts. The overall aim would be to empower children to deal with the road environment by giving them the requisite expertise, rather than merely exhorting them to 'behave safely'.

PSYCHOLOGICAL SKILLS REQUIRED TO INTERACT WITH TRAFFIC

The first attempts to analyse the road crossing task and its underlying functional processes were made by Older and Grayson (1974) and Avery (1974). These fairly general analyses were followed by a much more detailed examination by van der Molen (1981a), who used task analysis techniques to identify more than 200 sub-divisions of the pedestrian task. This study was partnered by an extremely influential paper by Vinjé (1981), who reviewed the functional capacities of young children in rela-tion to some of the key pedestrian tasks identified by van der Molen. In addition, she took the significant step of relating these capacities to developmental theory, specifically that of Jean Piaget. On the basis of this analysis, Vinjé listed a series of objectives which she considered viable with children of different ages, taking into account the capacities that could be assumed in each age group. She also suggested some simpler strategies that might be taught to younger children who would not have the ability to make more sophisticated judgements. We have extended this approach in the light of more recent research and theory in developmental psychology, focusing particularly on the extent to which underlying psychological skills might be promoted through educational intervention – a possibility that was never explored by earlier researchers (Thomson, 1991; Thomson et al., 1994). The following section summarises some of the key points of this analysis.

Detecting the presence of traffic

Obviously, pedestrians have to look for traffic in the first place if they are to avoid it. Having looked (in the sense of pointing their heads in the right direction), they also have to 'see' it. As we have noted, it is by no means obvious that children will, in fact, see traffic just because they have looked for it. Whether they do or not depends on the effectiveness of a number of underlying processes. First of all, an effective *visual search* strategy is required. This in turn depends on the pedestrian's conceptual representation of how cars move about the road environment – otherwise they would have no idea of where and where not to look, making their visual search inefficient. The pedestrian also requires the *attentional* capacity to focus on those cues that are relevant to the road crossing task and to ignore those that are irrelevant. Since irrelevant objects or events are frequently more interesting than relevant ones, there arises the problem of *distractibility* and how to counteract it. Additional factors influencing whether or not the pedestrian succeeds in detecting the presence of a vehicle include the accuracy of their *auditory localisation* and their ability to *co-ordinate* auditory and visual information. Finally, there are many circumstances on the road when an approaching vehicle *cannot* be seen and may not even be audible (e.g. when crossing near the brow of a hill, at a sharp bend, or near obstructing obstacles). Such locations are among the most dangerous on the road because the chances of detecting an approaching vehicle are greatly reduced from the outset: perhaps not surprisingly, such locations figure prominently in child accident statistics (Ampofo-Boateng and Thomson, 1991). It can be seen, then, that even detecting the presence of a vehicle depends on a number of primary perceptual and cognitive skills. If these are poorly developed, children may be placed in danger at the outset by simply failing to detect that there is a vehicle in the vicinity at all.

Visual timing judgements

Although detecting whether a vehicle is present or not turns out to be far more complex than might at first be thought, this represents only the first step in the process of crossing even a simple road. Once a vehicle has been detected, pedestrians must make a range of further judgements concerning the vehicle's movement. Firstly, they must detect if the vehicle is moving at all and, if so, in what direction. If there are vehicles on an approach path, then their *time-to-contact* with the pedestrian's proposed path across the road must be determined. These timing judgements are less important on quiet streets where the pedestrian might simply wait for the vehicle to pass. However, on many streets, to wait for the road to clear would mean waiting all day. On busier roads, it is vital that pedestrians learn to anticipate the size of oncoming gaps in the traffic, differentiating between those that are large enough to pass through safely and those that are not. These skills depend on the observer's sensitivity to a range of optical variables specifying time-to-contact, including distance and velocity information. Pedestrians must become attuned to the information afforded by such variables and learn how to co-ordinate their movements to them. Since everyone's movement characteristics are slightly different, this tuning must also be calibrated on an individual basis. Clearly, some form of practice is required in order to do this.

Co-ordinating information from different directions

There are few occasions where the pedestrian is required to deal with traffic approaching from a single direction, because traffic almost always approaches from at least two – and from three or four in the case of many intersections. This means that several judgements must be made and co-ordinated with each other before a crossing decision can be reached. Thus both *memory* and the ability to *divide attention* between tasks become important. Finally, all the information picked up has to be processed, and in rather a short time given the speed with which the road environment can change. This will depend on the speed and accuracy of the pedestrian's *information-processing*; the amount of *central processing capacity* available to do this; and especially, the effectiveness of the *strategies* which the pedestrian has developed to cope with a limited capacity system.

Co-ordinating perception and action

Finally, the perceptual judgements described above would be meaningless if made in isolation. For example, in order to decide whether it is possible to cross safely the pedestrian must relate the time *available* to the time *required* to cross. The latter is not constant but varies as a function of such factors as the width of the road and the pedestrian's own movement characteristics. Pedestrians need to know their movement capabilities (and limitations) and must be able to calibrate this with visual information about road width in order to anticipate the time they will need to cross that particular road. As adults, we are not normally aware of this calibration unless it changes, as when one temporarily becomes lame. In the elderly, the calibration may gradually change as movement becomes more restricted. Children, of course, must calibrate from scratch. The calibration must also be kept in tune and be updated as the child grows.

It can be seen, then, that even crossing a simple street involves a whole range of basic skills and capacities. In order to make safe and effective traffic judgements, the child must reach a certain level of competence in these skills. Teaching them might therefore seem to be a reasonable goal of road safety education. But road safety programmes in this country have never attempted to teach such skills. Instead, they have concentrated on general rules and guidelines – 'golden rules' like the Green Cross Code that are expected to hold good for the vast majority of traffic situations the child is likely to encounter. Nor has a systematic programme been developed that would allow the child to build on earlier skills in a progressive way, although this has long been advocated (e.g. Sheppard, 1975; Vinjé, 1981; Rothengatter, 1981). Perhaps it is hardly surprising that the benefits of traditional road safety education have been rather limited.

STRATEGIC ISSUES IN THE DEPLOYMENT OF SKILL AT THE ROADSIDE

In addition to developing competence in underlying perceptual and cognitive functions, the child must also learn how to deploy these appropriately in real traffic contexts. The distinction between *skill* and *strategy* is important. For example, a pedestrian might accurately assess the time-to-arrival of an approaching vehicle, yet make poor use of this information by leaving an inadequate safety margin when selecting a traffic gap to walk through. In fact, learning to deploy basic perceptual and cognitive capacities in a strategic way is one of the central processes in traffic education. There is no point in training basic psychological capacities in a vacuum. We cannot assume that children will know how to employ them appropriately at the roadside: they must learn how to do this.

How does one go about analysing issues of strategic planning? One obvious starting-point would be to compare the behaviour of groups who are known to have lower accident rates (i.e. adults) with those who are vulnerable (i.e. children) to see what the differences are. This would help us understand what adults do that makes them safer, whilst highlighting what children do that makes them vulnerable. This, in turn, would help determine what it is that children need to learn. The aim would be to make the vulnerable group behave more like the safe group, rather than inducing them to adhere to some purely theoretical notion of safe behaviour.

ADULT VERSUS CHILD BEHAVIOUR

A number of studies have, in fact, investigated the 'natural' road behaviour of adults and children, using unobtrusive observational methods (e.g. Howarth *et al.*, 1974; Grayson, 1975b; Routledge *et al.*, 1976; van der Molen, 1983; McLaren, 1993). The results prove extremely interesting. Although adults are many times less likely to be knocked down than children, this advantage does not arise as a result of greater willingness to adhere to what they have been taught about road safety. For example, although adults know the Green Cross Code (or the older Kerb Drill) quite well, their behaviour in traffic is simply nothing like that advocated by the Code. Adults do not stop at the kerb before crossing, as the Code advises; they do not wait for traffic to pass before stepping into the street; they do not walk directly across the road; they accept far tighter gaps in the traffic than any child would accept; and they even use the crown of the road as a 'half-way house', turning crossing into a two-stage process. In short, there is little correspondence between the injunctions of the Green Cross Code and adult behaviour. In spite of this, adults have many fewer accidents than children.

Children behave quite differently. They are much more likely than adults to stop at the kerb; they delay longer at the kerbside before attempting to cross; in general, they only accept large gaps in the traffic (sometimes only *very* large gaps); they are more likely to walk straight across the road; and they do not use the crown of the road as a half-way house. In short, adults do most of the things that the Green Cross Code tells them not to do, yet they are much safer on the road than children. How can this discrepancy be explained?

The discrepancy comes about because experienced road users adopt more sophisticated strategies than those taught by road safety education. Although contradicting the advice of the Green Cross Code, most of these strategies are not really examples of 'bad' behaviour. For example, the reason adults do not stop and look for traffic at the roadside is because *they assess the situation before arriving at the kerb in the first place*. This means there is no need to stop and they can cross without delay. The behaviour does not reflect carelessness or incompetence: rather, it reflects anticipation and skill. Similarly, the tendency of adults to step into the street before a vehicle has passed is a strategy that maximises the size of the gap into which they are stepping. This 'tucking in' is possible because adults look ahead for suitable gaps in the traffic. As soon as the leading car has passed they are ready to step out smartly, thereby making the gap to the next car as big as possible. This also means they can accept somewhat smaller gaps than would otherwise be the case. This is obviously useful on busier roads where large gaps might not often occur spontaneously.

Children, on the other hand, show none of this anticipation. In fact, children do not look for gaps at all. Instead, they look for cars and focus on them individually, in isolation. By examining cars one by one, the child fails to see the relationships between them and fails to examine them far enough ahead. They do not even consider whether the gap is big enough until the leading car has passed and by the time they get round to looking at the next one, the gap has dwindled. Children miss many perfectly safe opportunities to cross in this way. The problem seems to arise both from a lack of anticipation and from not knowing quite what they should be looking for at the roadside in the first place.

This shows that elementary strategies like the Green Cross Code are no more than a 'starter', suitable only for introducing children to the behaviour required to deal with very simple road situations. The Code does not provide an adequate strategy for dealing with more complex or busier roads and *everyone* abandons it sooner or later. Instead of thinking of the Code as a universal 'golden rule', a better approach would be to define a range of strategies suited to different road situations and to teach these progressively in accordance with the child's changing ability and experience.

The road safety researcher is thus in a dilemma because much road safety education seems rather too general to be really useful to the child. The fact that most of it is taught in the classroom as a series of verbal exercises means that it is also too abstract, failing to provide a meaningful context that can help promote understanding. Above all, it does not give children the opportunity to practise what has been preached or to learn from their errors – a crucial feature of learning anything at all. These criticisms are central but have never been addressed by road safety education.

PROBLEMS IN DEVISING ROAD CROSSING STRATEGIES FOR CHILDREN

What is the alternative? Should we perhaps simply teach children the more sophisticated adult strategies? Whilst recognising their positive attributes, obviously no one is going to advocate this. Encouraging children to adopt strategies such as stepping into the street before a car has passed, for instance, would be nothing short of criminally irresponsible. Children simply cannot be expected to cope with this degree of sophistication. Indeed, there is some evidence that the higher accident rates among boys may occur precisely because they do attempt to adopt adult-like strategies before they have the skills to sustain them (Foot, 1985; Thomson, 1991).

However, the correct course of action is not to begin telling children to start stepping into the street through narrow gaps in the traffic. It is to provide them with the skills and competences that will – eventually – enable them to deploy more advanced strategies safely. The problem is that, at present, children develop and test these skills on their own, on real roads, and without the benefit of any guidance whatever. Meanwhile, road safety education teaches only general rules and guidelines. Surely, this whole approach is misguided. Road safety training should provide children with the skills they really need in order to cope with traffic. Otherwise they will simply teach themselves, with all the accompanying hazards this necessarily implies.

What can be done?

Several approaches to this problem are possible. One is to simplify the more complex strategies used by adults so that they fall within the capabilities of children. These modified strategies, although simpler, might still be adequate given that children are usually exposed to less complex traffic situations in the first place. Moreover, it might be quite easy for children spontaneously to adapt these simpler strategies as their experience develops, making them better able to deal with more complex situations. This approach was first advocated by Vinjé (1981) and formed the basis of a long research programme at Groningen University which ultimately had a major effect on road safety education in the Netherlands (van der Molen, 1989).

A second approach would be to teach the skills that underlie the more mature strategies used by adults. This should help bring about the conditions in which more efficient strategies become possible. For example, to reach a stage where pedestrians can differentiate between traffic gaps, they must acquire the underlying visual timing skills. This approach, emphasising the importance of developing the basic perceptual and cognitive skills that underlie strategic planning, has been particularly strongly advocated by our group at Strathclyde University (Thomson, 1991; Thomson *et al.*, 1994). The reason is that, unless children fully understand what underlies the strategy, there is a very strong risk that they will apply it rigidly and inappropriately. We have already commented on the inappropriate ways in which children sometimes use the Green Cross Code. It is therefore essential that any rules or strategies are accompanied by matching conceptual development so that the child understands the purpose behind the rule. Only in this way can we expect the rules to be applied intelligently.

Finally, it might be possible to find ways of developing basic competences *and* strategic planning at the same time. This would be useful, because it would ensure that children's strategic thinking about traffic would evolve as part of their developing skill base. A number of examples of this approach can be found in recent research, although little has yet found its way into the standard road safety education that children in the UK are likely to receive. However, this situation is rapidly changing as both central and local government become increasingly aware of these alternatives to traditional approaches. It is to these alternatives that we now turn.

ADAPTING PEDESTRIAN STRATEGIES FOR CHILDREN

Simple road crossing

The most obvious example of a pedestrian strategy designed for children is the Green Cross Code, whose characteristics we have already discussed. The behavioural elements advocated by the Code are perfectly sensible in relation to crossing simple, quiet streets. However, it is an elementary strategy and not well suited to more complex traffic situations. This is a problem, because the Code is generally assumed to be the definitive way to cross the road in any situation. In addition, it has at least one major weakness in failing to recognise the difficulty children have in finding safe places to cross. This renders them vulnerable from the very outset, no matter how carefully they try to put the other precepts of the Code into practice.

Nevertheless, if its limitations are recognised, the Code does offer an introduction to the elements of road crossing for the very young child. A carefully constructed road safety training programme designed to build on this could gradually improve the child's competence. Unfortunately, no such systematic attempts are made in this country. Moreover, because of its verbal nature the Code is not suitable for most children under 7–8 years of age. This means that younger children are taught the even more general Stop, Look, Listen, Think strategy, which is even less clear about what children should do in concrete traffic situations.

However, when taught in a behavioural way at the roadside, there is good reason to believe that even very young children can learn to use the Code effectively and can remember how to do so over a period of time. Rothengatter (1981) taught a strategy very similar to the Green Cross Code (known in the Netherlands as the Basic Strategy) using a behavioural modelling technique based on the principles of social learning theory (Bandura, 1977). When taught in a roadside context, children as young as 4 years of age showed considerable competence in crossing and retained that competence several months later. By contrast, when taught as a verbal rule, it is not even possible to begin training until several years later. Few examples more clearly illustrate the benefits of a practical approach over a verbal one.

Strategies for more complex traffic situations

This basic strategy represents no more than the first in a series of strategies that children must acquire if they are to deal with the range of problems posed by the road environment. An example is crossing near parked cars – a situation that, as we saw in the previous chapter, is associated with a large number of child pedestrian accidents (Demetre and Gaffin, 1994). One way of dealing with the problem would be to teach children to avoid crossing near parked cars altogether. In practice, however, this would be rather pious advice since in many areas it is often impossible to avoid them. In any case, it is actually possible to cross safely near parked vehicles so long as an appropriate strategy is adopted. This involves choosing a suitable space between the parked vehicles; checking that one of them is not about to move off (e.g. that they are unoccupied, that reversing or other lights are not on, that there are no exhaust fumes, etc.); and stopping appropriately at the line of sight (the outer edge of the car). The steps needed to cross near parked vehicles are essentially an elaboration of the Basic Strategy, so if taught to children who have already learned how to cross where the road is clear, the parked car strategy is mastered relatively easily. A systematic strategy was first developed by Rothengatter (1981) which has recently been elaborated by our group for use in a UK context (Thomson, 1995). In both countries, children as young as 5–6 years of age can learn to use it appropriately after a small number (4–6) of training sessions.

Further strategies can be evolved for other traffic situations, such as crossing at junctions. As with parked cars, junctions are heavily implicated in accidents, especially in younger children (e.g. Howarth *et al.*, 1974; van Schagen, 1985). It seems obvious that they should learn what is dangerous about such locations and how to deal with them. Again, a strategy for doing so can be developed and effectively trained in children as young as 6–7 years of age (Rothengatter, 1981; van Schagen, 1985; Thomson, 1995). In this way, identifying dangerous road situations and learning how to deal with them represents a concrete way forward in the process of preparing children to face the road environment.

PROMOTING SKILL DEVELOPMENT IN CHILDREN

The above approach has many admirable features, particularly in the stress laid on practical training. However, a number of difficulties remain. For example, the Basic Strategy, like the Green Cross Code, does not teach children how to recognise a dangerous place or how to find a safer one where the strategy could be put into practice. This problem is to some extent dealt with in later parts of the programme where parked vehicle and intersection strategies are taught. However, we have argued that the ability to find a safe place logically precedes the need for a crossing strategy because, if children cannot discriminate safe from dangerous places, there is the strong possibility that they will use their crossing routine inappropriately. Thus, the learning of a routine for crossing should never be dissociated from the skills that underlie it.

Ideally, then, we need training which develops basic skills as well as teaching strategies. Let us consider two skills which have been taught in this way. They are worth considering because of their importance in road behaviour and also because they have now received a good deal of analysis and investigation.

Visual timing skills

The first example concerns the visual timing skills to which we have already referred, which are clearly central to safe pedestrian behaviour. However, no current road safety programme attempts to teach these. The Green Cross Code, for example, simply instructs the child to wait until the road is clear before crossing. Such advice may be appropriate for the very young pedestrian who, as we have seen, deals primarily with quiet roads. However, on many roads it is quite impracticable to wait for the road to clear completely. Moreover, children have a tendency to interpret instructions such as 'wait until the road clears' very literally. We have seen children interpret this so literally that they were unwilling to cross if they could see a car at all. This degree of rigidity is not functional and suggests that the children were not just being conservative about safety but were blindly following a rule. It is obvious that at some time they must start crossing in a more efficient manner, accepting gaps in the traffic that are safe to move through whilst rejecting those that are not. We might argue about the age at which such training should begin but it hardly seems sensible to refuse to train children in such skills at all. The problem is to find ways of teaching them in a safe but effective manner. Since they involve fundamentally practical judgements, it is hard to see how they could be learned without 'hands-on' experience. On the other hand, we can scarcely ask children to practise in real traffic: a safe but realistic alternative must be found.

An intriguing way of doing this was devised by Lee and his collaborators at Edinburgh University (Lee *et al.*, 1984; Young and Lee, 1987; Demetre *et al.*, 1992, 1993). The method involves setting up a 'pretend road' next to a real one as shown in Figure 7.1. The child observes traffic passing on the real road but crosses the adjacent pretend one. Thus, their visual judgements are natural, as is their behaviour when trying to cross. However, no harm comes to them if they make errors: in fact, errors provide feedback and promote learning. The method thus offers controlled experience of making roadside judgements about dynamic traffic situations. Moreover, the situations can be made simple or complex simply by selecting appropriate roads to practise by. This basic method has been investigated in a number of more recent studies in which the paradigm has been varied to explore the nature of children's judgements in such contexts (e.g. van Schagen, 1988; Demetre *et al.*, 1992, 1993).

The main measures of crossing performance that have been derived in such studies are:

- *Tight fits* These are defined as gaps in the traffic which the child thinks are large enough to pass through but which are, in fact, too small to allow them to reach the opposite kerb before the car passes. The child would not necessarily be knocked down in such a situation (adults also

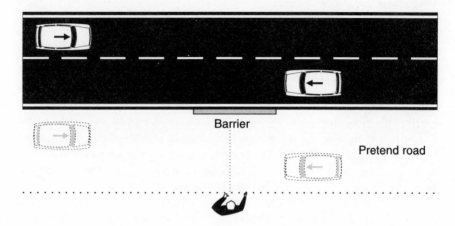

Figure 7.1 The pretend road crossing task

Source: From Lee *et al.*, 1984; Young and Lee, 1987; Demetre *et al.*, 1992, 1993

have tight fits because they allow cars to pass behind them whilst they are still on the road) but the behaviour is clearly dangerous and should be discouraged.

- *Missed opportunities* These occur when the child rejects gaps that could be safely passed through. The definition of what constitutes a missed opportunity varies from study to study but, when the vehicle is in the nearside lane, a missed opportunity is usually defined as a gap of more than one and a half times the time it would take to cross the entire road. In practice, children tend to reject gaps that are far larger than this.
- *Crossing time* This measures how long the child needs to cross a particular road. It is essential in defining other measures, such as missed opportunities.
- *Starting delay* This measures how smartly the child steps out after the leading car has passed. It reflects perceptual anticipation and the extent to which the child is looking ahead for suitable gaps, as opposed to just watching the cars pass one by one.

There are very clear developmental trends on such tests, with younger children (aged 5–8) making too many tight fits on the one hand, and missing many opportunities to cross in safety on the other. Often, children will reject really large gaps, thereby appearing very conservative in their judgements. However, the same children will, from time to time, accept a tight fit where they would definitely be in danger if crossing a real road. The behaviour of inexperienced child pedestrians is often erratic in this way, as has often been pointed out by road safety researchers (e.g.

Sandels, 1975). Older children make more mature judgements, being less likely to miss safe opportunities to cross but also being less likely to accept tight fits. These trends can be seen in Figure 7.2, which shows the size of gaps that children of different ages and adults are willing to accept on the pretend road. (It also shows what adults do on real roads). It can be seen that adults accept almost no gaps of less than about 4 seconds. At the same time, they accept almost all those of more than about 6 or 7 seconds. In other words, they have a very small area of uncertainty about what constitutes a safe gap and what does not. By contrast, younger children reject a large number of perfectly safe gaps (e.g. only about 30 per cent of 10 second gaps are accepted). On the other hand, they also accept a small number of gaps that are far too short and which could definitely not be passed through safely. This occasionally includes gaps of less than 2 seconds. Clearly, these children require experience of making traffic judgements.

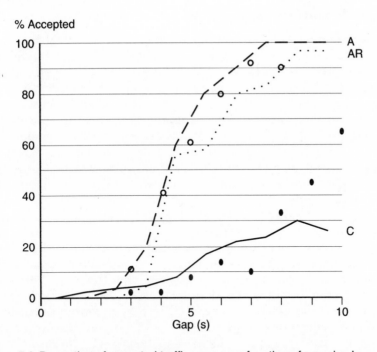

Figure 7.2 Proportion of accepted traffic gaps as a function of gap size by children (C) and adults (A) in pretend road crossing and by adults (AR) in real road crossing.

Source: From Lee *et al.*, 1984

Note: Open and filled circles are data for normal road crossing obtained by unobtrusive observation (replotted from Routledge *et al.*, 1976, Figure 1). Open circles = adults; filled circles = 5–9 year-olds.

Following training, however, the picture changes substantially, even in children as young as 5 years of age. For example, Young and Lee (1987) found that, following about six half-hour training sessions, children's crossing times became more stable; they missed far fewer safe opportunities to cross; and, significantly, they did not generate more tight fits in the process. Thus, the children were not just 'going earlier' in a rigid sort of way: they were improving their timing skills and were applying them appropriately.

This approach to road safety education would appear to have much to offer. In giving children experience of making traffic judgements in a realistic but controlled way they have the opportunity both to improve their basic timing skills *and* to deploy these skills effectively. There is no clear separation between skill and strategy in this paradigm because both are tackled simultaneously. This seems an ideal way to formulate training.

Constructing safe routes through the road environment

Another example that combines the training of fundamental skills with strategic deployment comes from our own research at Strathclyde University where we have been concerned with children's perception of danger and their ability to construct safe routes through the road environment (e.g. Ampofo-Boateng and Thomson, 1991; Thomson *et al.*, 1992; Ampofo-Boateng *et al.*, 1993). This approach arose from the finding that certain roadside locations are intrinsically more dangerous than others and are over-represented in child accident statistics. Examples include places of reduced visibility (e.g. near obstructions like parked vehicles, sharp bends, the brow of a hill, etc.) and places where traffic moves in multiple directions (intersections, roundabouts, etc.). Such locations should either be avoided altogether or the pedestrian needs a special strategy for dealing with them.

Unfortunately, young children do not appreciate that such locations are dangerous in the first place, and they will readily choose to cross there if given the opportunity (Ampofo-Boateng and Thomson, 1991). It is surprising how insensitive children are to such dangers, which appear very obvious to adults. The problem is that children can appreciate that a situation is dangerous when vehicles are visibly present. However, they find it much harder to appreciate that situations can be dangerous when vehicles are visibly *absent*: or, more correctly, that vehicles can be present when they *appear to be absent*. In fact, if cars are visible young children will always judge the situation dangerous and will refuse to cross the road. However, if they cannot see cars children almost always think the situation is safe. Thus, positions such as a sharp, occluded bend or the brow of a hill are considered to be perfectly safe by most children under the age of about 9 years. Only older children realise that such sites are dangerous precisely because no traffic can be seen.

Existing countermeasures have not recognised this as a problem at all. For example, the Green Cross Code simply instructs children to 'first find a safe place', which assumes that they can do so. The problem is fundamental because, if children attempt to cross at a blind summit, they will be in danger no matter how well they have mastered the Green Cross Code or even the more sophisticated timing skills discussed above. For this reason, children should be taught how to recognise such dangerous locations *before* they learn the crossing strategies that are the main focus of almost all current road safety education.

Can these skills be taught? We have recently attempted to answer this question by devising a training programme for 5 year-olds, aimed at bringing their performance closer to the level of older, more experienced pedestrians (Thomson *et al.*, 1992; Ampofo-Boateng *et al.*, 1993). Children were trained either individually or in small groups either at the roadside or using table-top models of traffic scenes where situations similar to those at the roadside could be contrived. The children were tested prior to training (to obtain a baseline measure of their skill); and were retested at several different times during the six months after training ended. We also compared their judgements to those of age-matched children who had received no training at all.

In all the permutations of this experiment, the results showed a substantial improvement after training, with the proportion of children making 'safe' responses rising substantially. The degree of improvement varied according to whether children were trained individually or in groups, with individually-trained children making the largest immediate gains. However, after a two month delay, the performances of individually and group-trained children had more or less equalised. About 40 per cent of the routes chosen by trained children were deemed to be safe as against only 12 per cent before training began, an improvement of nearly 350 per cent. This placed 5 year-olds closer to the performance of untrained 9 year-olds than to that of control 5 year-old children. Interestingly, there was no difference between those trained by the combined real world/model condition and those trained entirely in the real world. From this we can infer that a realistic simulation, at least when combined with an element of real-world training, can improve children's roadside judgements. The use of such simulations should be further investigated.

It would appear, then, that it is possible to train this type of skill even in very young children and to produce improvements over a fairly short period of time. Our training consisted of only six sessions of about half an hour each, at a rate of one a week. In spite of this modest amount of training, quite marked benefits were obtained and much of this was

maintained over a considerable period following the end of the programme. It should be stressed that safe place finding is a conceptually
challenging problem for young children and is certainly not just a matter
of stringing rules together. What improved after training was, in fact,
children's *reasoning* about the factors that render locations safe or dangerous. This produced a substantial improvement in the safety of the routes
they constructed on the basis of that reasoning.

Summary

These studies show that children as young as 4–5 years of age can be
taught to make traffic judgements more like those of experienced pedestrians, provided appropriate training methods are used. By contrast to
traditional approaches based on knowledge enhancement, it would appear that practical training has a good deal to offer, with even complex
skills being amenable to training. There is certainly no evidence to
support the view that children cannot learn such skills before a certain
developmental stage has been reached. The critical issue seems to be the
methods that are adopted and the sort of experience that these provide.

The real advantage of practical training is that it provides a meaningful
context within which training can take place. Children are thus not required to 'pretend' they are at the roadside when they are, in fact, sitting
in the classroom. Nor are they asked to infer what would happen if they
were to do such-and-such, because they can *see* what happens. They thus
receive immediate and appropriate feedback which promotes learning.
The importance of conducting training in the correct context is likely to be
much more important for younger children, who have not yet developed
a strong conceptual model of the traffic environment. Outwith that context they are almost bound to have difficulty in understanding what the
trainer is talking about when asked to think about one context when they
are, in fact, in another (Thomson *et al.*, 1994). Ironically, insofar as children receive practical experience at all, it is much more likely to be with
older children, who are less in need of it.

PROBLEMS OF IMPLEMENTING PRACTICAL ROAD SAFETY TRAINING

It is apparent that practical training has the potential to increase the
accuracy and effectiveness of children's traffic judgements. Unfortunately
practical methods give rise to practical problems, for such methods are
intrinsically time consuming and labour intensive. Even given the
progress that can be made with 4–6 training sessions each lasting only
half an hour, this still represents a considerable load given current

resources. This is by far the biggest problem facing anyone thinking of introducing such methods on a large scale. The question is, who can be expected to undertake such training?

RSTOs and the police

At present, road safety training is primarily the responsibility of Road Safety Training Officers employed by local authorities (although the police continue to make an important contribution through their programmes of school visits). Individual RSTOs typically have responsibility for a very large number of schools in their area and it is therefore not their primary role to work directly with individual children. It is certainly unrealistic to expect that RSTOs would themselves undertake front-line practical training of children. Their role would lie mainly in preparing other people to undertake such work and to provide them with the materials and expertise needed to do so effectively. There remains the question as to who these 'other people' should be.

The role of the school

Most RSTOs spend a significant amount of their time promoting road safety education in schools by making resource materials available and by helping teachers decide how the subject can be built into the curriculum in a beneficial manner. It might therefore be asked whether teachers could not add at least an element of practical training to the road safety education that they already undertake.

Most schools certainly seem to feel that they should play some part in road safety education but it must be recognised that, in general, they do not seem to feel that their role should be a pivotal one (Foot *et al.*, 1982; Singh, 1982). In practice, there is very wide variation both in the amount and content of the road safety education that schools provide and most operate without any clear cut policy on the issue (Singh and Speare, 1989). There is also much variation in how the subject figures in the curriculum: for example, as a subject in its own right versus integrated across the curriculum. Nevertheless, many resources aimed at teachers and the school have been developed including, in recent years, practical training packages aimed at fostering skills of the sort discussed above. For example, a recently developed package showing how training in the identification of roadside dangers can be promoted through traffic trails in the streets near the school and through classroom exercises using table-top models, has been obtained by many local authorities across the UK. Although the package has been evaluated with positive results (Tucker, 1993), it remains to be seen how widespread its use will actually be.

Nevertheless, such resources enable the school to provide at least some practical experience of traffic to children. It seems likely that further efforts in this direction will be made.

Nevertheless, there is a limit to what the school can be expected to contribute on its own, particularly given the substantial burden that teachers already bear in relation to an ever-increasing range of activities. There appears to be a tendency to view the school as the natural home for virtually any activity that can be construed as having an educational element. Whilst there is obviously a grain of truth in this, one has to be realistic about what else can simply be passed across to teachers to deal with. Whilst many teachers might well succeed in integrating an element of practical road safety education into their timetable, this is most likely to be on an occasional basis and therefore to fall short of what is being proposed here. Even 4–6 sessions at the roadside, especially when working with children in small groups, simply means too many trips for a class teacher to be expected to cope alone. Once again, an input from elsewhere is required.

The role of parents

Of all those groups who might be expected to contribute something to road safety education, it is parents who tend to be considered as bearing primary responsibility – a view largely shared by parents themselves (Sadler, 1972; Foot et al., 1982). Whether this view is entirely fair is, in our opinion, debatable. It goes without saying that parents are more concerned about their children's safety than anyone else, and it follows naturally that they will feel a corresponding responsibility to do something about it. However, substantial obligations also lie with the rest of society who plan the road environment (usually with little thought for the needs of pedestrians); who drive around it; and who benefit from the existence of traffic in diverse ways. Child safety is a problem of society as a whole and society needs to realise that the benefits it derives from traffic are accompanied by risks which, for children, outweigh the risks they are likely to suffer from any other source.

Nevertheless, parents certainly have more opportunities to train their children than anyone else, particularly when it comes to providing practical experience (which they can give in the context of simple everyday activities like going to the shops), and it seems foolish to reject this 'resource'. It is therefore worth exploring what role parents might realistically be expected to play in the process of road safety education and what resources they would need in order to do so.

There is certainly little point in merely exhorting parents to teach road safety and then just hoping for the best. Although more concerned about their children's safety than anyone else, the fact is many parents simply have no clear idea of what to teach and often have little confidence in themselves as teachers. Moreover, it appears that parents may quite seriously misjudge what their children are capable of doing. For example, Sadler (1972) interviewed a sample of over 2000 mothers and found that 25 per cent of them had introduced their children to only one or two specific roads by the time they were 8 years old. By contrast to this very conservative approach, almost 20 per cent had introduced children as young as 3 years to 'very busy' roads and 13 per cent regarded their 2 year-old children as capable of crossing such a road unaided! While this degree of optimism is extreme, there will be few readers who have not come across examples of very young children running errands that required them to cross streets unaided. Clearly, many parents need guidance as to what their children are capable of, as well as what they themselves can do to improve on this.

Traffic clubs

Most countries, including the UK, have attempted to involve parents in their children's road safety education, usually through the distribution of booklets and similar materials. However, a more systematic approach was taken by the Scandinavian Traffic Club which produced dedicated materials for parents and sent these out on a regular (six-monthly) basis. A marked feature of the Norwegian club was that it strongly encouraged parents to carry out practical exercises with their children. The most superficially impressive result was that accident rates were found to be 20 per cent lower amongst club members relative to non-members, a difference that was even more marked in the only major urban conurbation in the country (Oslo). The children's road safety knowledge was also superior. These findings have led to the introduction of similar schemes elsewhere in Scandinavia as well as in West Germany and Luxembourg. The idea of a national traffic club has been piloted in the Eastern Region of England, with reasonably encouraging results (West, Sammons and West, 1993). However, this club focused on elementary road safety education among very young children.

Two notes of caution need to be sounded with regard to the success of such traffic clubs, however. Firstly, with regard to the Norwegian experiment, the observed decline in accident rates was not accompanied by any discernible changes in the road behaviour of member children. That is, there was no evidence that members were behaving more safely in traffic than non-members (Schioldborg, 1974, 1976). This raises the possibility that the reduced accident rates were, in some way, an artefact. Since membership of the club was voluntary and only a third to a half of eligible children actually joined, it is possible that the parents who enrolled their children were safety conscious in the first place and that their children were less likely to have a road accident whether they joined the club or not. Another possibility is that member parents became increasingly safety conscious as a result of participating in the study and became more protective towards their children for this reason. The observed differences in accident rates would thus reflect differences in *exposure* between the two groups, not differences in traffic skill as a result of undergoing the programme. Whilst possibly desirable in itself, changes in exposure would not represent a fulfilment of the stated aims of the programme and it would certainly not contribute to the long-term preparation of children for independent travel.

The second note of caution is that, as we have seen, only a proportion of eligible parents actually take part in traffic clubs – a proportion which, in the case of the Norwegian experiment, was less than half. Moreover, membership tends to be biased towards higher socio-economic groups (Downing, 1981), whereas it is well known that accidents are over-represented among lower socio-economic groups. Some means therefore needs to be found of increasing the participation of parents from lower socio-economic backgrounds, or ensuring in some other way that children from accident-prone communities receive training. The notion of a traffic club is a good one, because it gives parents far clearer guidance than they would otherwise receive as to what they can do to improve their children's traffic competence. However, if such approaches are to fulfil their potential some way needs to be found of increasing participation, particularly among the more vulnerable sections of the community.

Community-based approaches to road safety education

An approach that we have been piloting is to set up a community-based Road Safety Initiative in which parent volunteers work in collaboration with local schools and the Initiative staff (Thomson *et al.*, 1993, 1995). A critical aspect is that the volunteers receive guided instruction as to how children should be trained at a course organised by the project staff, rather than indirectly through books and pamphlets sent through the post. A second critical feature is that volunteers are not asked to train their own children. Rather, they are asked to participate in a training programme aimed at *all* children in a particular year group, by taking responsibility for small groups of children who are assigned to them on a random basis. In this way, all the children benefit, not just those whose own parents feel capable of making the required commitment. The approach is thus fundamentally focused on *community action*, aimed at improving child safety within the community as a whole, and not just on 'local' action within the family. So far as we know, no such approach to road safety education has ever before been taken.

The approach has a number of advantages over alternatives. Firstly, it ensures that a large number of children come in contact with the scheme and benefit from it. In this way, the biases referred to above are eliminated. Secondly, the volunteers constitute a substantial resource and their participation greatly increases the amount of practical training that children can receive. In our case, volunteers were asked to train the children in groups of two or three (depending on the skill), collecting them directly from the classroom and returning them afterwards. This means that, over a period of six weeks (the usual length of our training programme), children received a substantial amount of practical experience without this increasing the workload of teachers at all. Thirdly, the training programme focused on a set of clearly defined pedestrian skills whose absence is known to be associated with risk (safe place finding; crossing at parked cars; and crossing at junctions). None of these would be easy to teach without practical training. Finally, the programme helps to improve contact between parents and the school more generally – a desirable objective in itself.

This research project is not yet complete but it is already quite clear that parents, even those from vulnerable communities, can substantially increase their children's traffic competence. Indeed, it is surprising how successful parents can be in this. Figure 7.3 shows the results obtained by a group of 10 parents from a vulnerable part of Glasgow who had volunteered to train children in how to recognise dangerous places on the road and construct safe routes that avoided them (Thomson *et al.*, 1993). The figure shows the proportion of routes chosen by the children that could be considered safe before they were trained (pre-test); immediately after training (post-test 1); and after a further two month delay during which they received no training (post-test 2). The results are shown relative to those obtained in an earlier study where children were trained by 'experts' (Thomson *et al.*, 1992).

It can be seen that, in this sample at least, there was no difference between experts and parent volunteers in the effectiveness of their training. Indeed, the parents performed marginally better. The situations are not quite comparable, because the parental volunteers trained children in groups of three whereas the experts trained in groups of five which is obviously more demanding. Even allowing for this, the success of the volunteers is striking. Nor had these parents any special qualifications for undertaking such work, other than an interest in the welfare of children and being parents themselves. The results suggest that parents from deprived and accident-prone areas of major cities may be able to contribute substantially to the road safety education of local children, provided they themselves have been trained and clearly appreciate what they are supposed to be doing and why. It remains to be seen whether larger scale studies will confirm these trends. However, our research leads us to be optimistic about the likely outcome.

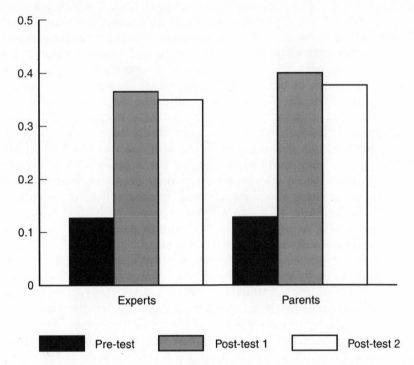

Figure 7.3 Proportion of 'safe' routes across the road constructed by 5 year-old children before and after training by either 'experts' or parent volunteers.

Source: Thomson *et al.*, 1993

CONCLUSIONS

A number of conclusions may be drawn from this chapter, all of which have implications for road safety education. They concern everything from the content of current provision to who should be responsible for providing it. The proposed answers, if followed, would carry road safety education in a quite different direction from that taken over the last thirty years or so.

1 The first proposal is that, in order to cope effectively with modern traffic, pedestrians must have competence in a whole range of basic perceptual and cognitive skills. They must also be able to deploy these skills appropriately across a wide range of traffic contexts. Road safety education needs to make a far greater effort to identify these skills and competences and to produce educational packages that improve them in concrete and clearly defined ways. Too much road safety education

starts with vague and ill-defined objectives such as 'improving child-ren's understanding of traffic', 'helping children to behave safely' or even 'reducing accidents'. All these aims are perfectly laudable but are far too vague to be helpful to the designer of an educational package: what exactly is meant by ' behave safely', for instance? In order to achieve such general objectives, it is necessary to break them down into a set of far more specific, concrete objectives and show why training in these should lead, progressively, to attainment of the overall goal. Unfortunately road safety education has not, on the whole, paid great attention to the problems of defining educational objectives. As we noted earlier, there seems to be an implicit view that, if the material deals with road safety at all, then it is almost bound to be beneficial. The evidence is simply not consistent with such a view.

2 Although most road safety education is concerned with enhancing children's knowledge about traffic and their attitudes to safety, there is little evidence that such approaches have any effect on the way child-ren behave in traffic. This is by far the most serious criticism of current road safety provision as a whole. At one level, we should not be unduly surprised by this. Road crossing is a practical skill and the best way to learn it is by doing it, not talking about it. Of course, the learning must take place in a safe and controlled environment so that the children learn from their errors rather than die from them. In this chapter we have described a number of ways in which such practical experience can be given.

3 The critical issue is, who can be expected to undertake such training? Although a wide range of agencies now regard themselves as having a role to play in accident reduction (Ward, 1991), it is surprisingly hard to determine who should be responsible for what and how inter-agency co-operation can be assured. It seems likely that this will remain an issue for some considerable time. Perhaps it is not surprising that Singh (1982) described children's road safety as 'everyone's concern but no-one's responsibility'.

In the end, road safety education always seems to come down to parents and the school, albeit with the support of a network of RSTOs and the police. If practical training is to be introduced on the necessary scale, it must draw on these resources. In this chapter, we have discussed possible ways of preparing them for the task, including the kinds of support they will need in order to be effective. We have also discussed the possibility of a more innovative approach based on community action rather than purely parent action. Of course, this approach requires organisation and the implicit support of a wide range of agencies including teachers, the school, local authority departments and the police. Nevertheless, our experience is that such co-operation is possible when a clearly defined programme of action is proposed. The approach is particularly appealing in that it goes some way towards acknowledging the obligations of the wider society in which children live to their safety. In our experience, many vulnerable communities are intensely aware of the threat facing their children and are highly motivated to do something about it (cf. also Chapter 4 on accidents in the home and at play). Increased efforts should be made to find ways of enabling communities to participate in such enterprises and to contribute to their own, and their children's, safety.

REFERENCES

Ampofo-Boateng, K. and Thomson, J. A. (1991) 'Children's perception of safety and danger on the road', *British Journal of Psychology* 82: 487–505.

Ampofo-Boateng, K., Thomson, J. A., Grieve, R., Pitcairn, T., Lee, D. N. and Demetre, J. D. (1993) 'A developmental and training study of children's ability to find safe routes to cross the road', *British Journal of Developmental Psychology* 11: 31–45.

Avery, G. C. (1974) 'The capacity of young children to cope with the traffic system: a review', Traffic Accident Research Unit, Department of Motor Transport, New South Wales, Australia.

Bandura, A. (1977) *Social Learning Theory*, Englewood Cliffs: Prentice-Hall.

Davies, J., Guy, J. and Murray, G. (1993) 'You decide to stay alive: a child pedestrian project, years 1–3', Transport Research Laboratory Report PR/SRC/15/9, Crowthorne: TRL.

Demetre, J. D., Lee, D. N., Pitcairn, T. K., Grieve, R., Thomson, J. A. and Ampofo-Boateng, K. (1992) 'Errors in young children's decisions about traffic gaps: experiments with roadside simulations', *British Journal of Psychology* 83: 189–202.

Demetre, J. D., Lee, D. N., Grieve, R., Pitcairn, T. K., Ampofo-Boateng, K. and Thomson, J. A. (1993) 'Young children's learning on road-crossing simulations', *British Journal of Educational Psychology* 63: 348–58.

Demetre, J. D. and Gaffin, S. (1994) 'The salience of occluding vehicles to child pedestrians', *British Journal of Educational Psychology* 64: 243–51.

Downing, C. S. (1981) 'Improving parental road safety practice and education with respect to pre-school children', in H. C. Foot, A. J. Chapman and F. M. Wade (eds) *Road Safety: Research and Practice*, Eastbourne: Praeger.

Foot, H. C. (1985) 'Boys will be boys?', *Safety Education* 1: 1–6.

Foot, H. C., Chapman, A. J. and Wade, F. M. (1982) 'Pedestrian accidents: issues and approaches', in A. J. Chapman, F. M. Wade and H. C. Foot (eds) *Pedestrian Accidents*, Chichester: John Wiley.

Grayson, G. B. (1975a) 'The Hampshire child pedestrian accident study', Department of the Environment Report 670, Crowthorne: TRRL.

Grayson, G. B. (1975b) 'Observations of pedestrians at four sites', Department of the Environment Report 670, Crowthorne: TRRL.

Howarth, C. I., Routledge, D. A. and Repetto-Wright, R. (1974) 'An analysis of road accidents involving young children', *Ergonomics* 17: 319–30.

Lee, D. N., Young, D. S. and McLaughlin, C. M. (1984) 'A roadside simulation of road crossing for young children', *Ergonomics* 2, 1271–81.

McLaren, B. D. (1993) 'An observational study of behavioural sex differences in adult road crossing skill', unpublished master's dissertation, University of Strathclyde.

Molen, H. H. van der (1981a) 'Blueprint of an analysis of the pedestrian task-1. Method of analysis', *Accident Analysis and Prevention* 13: 175–91.

—— (1981b) 'Child pedestrian's exposure, accidents and behaviour', *Accident Analysis and Prevention* 13: 193–224.

—— (1983) 'Pedestrian ethology', doctoral dissertation, University of Groningen, Netherlands.

—— (1989) 'World pedestrian training: experience and possibilities for world wide application', *World Safety Journal* 111: 23–5.

MVA Consultancy (1989) *Must Do Better: A Study of Child Pedestrian Accidents and Road Crossing Behaviour in Scotland*, Scottish Office, Central Research Unit Papers. Edinburgh: Scottish Development Department.

Older, S. J. and Grayson, G. B. (1974) 'Perception and decision in the pedestrian task', Department of the Environment Report 49UC, Crowthorne: TRRL.

Rothengatter, J. A. (1981) *Traffic Safety Education for Young Children*, Lisse: Swets and Reitlinger.

Rothengatter, T. (1984) 'A behavioural approach to improving traffic behaviour of young children', *Ergonomics* 2: 147–60.

Routledge, D. A., Howarth, C. I. and Repetto-Wright, R. (1976) 'The development of road crossing skill by child pedestrians', in A. S. Hakkert, *Proceedings of the International Conference on Road Safety Vol. 1*, Haifa: Michlol Technion.

Sadler, J. (1972) *Children and Road Safety: A Survey Amongst Mothers*, London: HMSO.

Sandels, S. (1975) *Children in Traffic*, London: Elek.

Schagen, van I. (1985) 'Crossing at junctions: experimental application of a road safety module for primary schools', in R. A. de Bruin (ed.) *Traffic Research Centre Annual Report 1985*, University of Gronigen: Netherlands.

Schagen, van I. (1988) 'Training children to make safe crossing decisions', in J. A. Rothengatter and R. A. de Bruin (eds) *Road User Behaviour: Theory and Practice*, Assen: Van Gorum.

Schioldborg, P. (1974) 'Children, traffic and traffic training: an analysis of the children's traffic club', unpublished report, Psychological Institute, University of Oslo, Norway.

Schioldborg, P. (1976) 'Children, traffic and traffic training', paper presented at the Fifth Congress of the International Federation of Pedestrians, Geilo, Norway.

Scottish Development Department (1989) 'Must do better: a study of child pedestrian accidents and road crossing behaviour in Scotland', Scottish Office, Central Research Unit Papers, Edinburgh: Scottish Development Department.

Sheppard, D. (1975) 'Teaching pedestrian skills: a graded structure', *Safety Education* 133: 5–7.

Singh, A. (1982) 'Pedestrian education', in A. J. Chapman, F. M. Wade and H. C. Foot (eds) *Pedestrian Accidents*, Chichester: John Wiley.

Singh, A. and Speare, M. (1989) 'Road Safety Education in Schools and Colleges', Transport and Road Research Laboratory Report 133, Crowthorne: TRRL.

Thomson, J. A. (1991) *The Facts about Child Pedestrian Accidents*, London: Cassell.

—— (1995) 'The effectiveness of a community-based approach to road safety education using practical training methods: the Drumchapel project', Report to Strathclyde Regional Council, Department of Roads.

Thomson, J. A., Ampofo-Boateng, K., Pitcairn, T., Grieve, R., Lee, D. N. and Demetre, J. D. (1992) 'Behavioural group training of children to find safe routes to cross the road', *British Journal of Educational Psychology* 62: 173–83.

Thomson, J. A., Lee, D. N., Pitcairn, T. K., Grieve, R., Ampofo-Boateng, K. and Demetre, J. D. (1993) 'Development of pedestrian skills in young children by means of practical training', in Grayson, G. (ed.) *Behavioural Research on Road Safety III*, Crowthorne: TRL.

Thomson, J. A., Tolmie, A. K., Foot, H. C. and McLaren, B. (1994) 'Child pedestrian accidents from the perspective of developmental psychology: a review and analysis', Report to the Department of Transport (to be published by HMSO).

Tucker, S. (1993) 'A pedestrian training resource for children aged 5 to 8', Transport Research Laboratory Report PR/SRC/16/93, Crowthorn: TRL.

Vinjé, M. P. (1981) 'Children as pedestrians: abilities and limitations', *Accident Analysis and Prevention* 13, 225–40.

Ward, H. (1991) *Preventing Road Accidents to Children: The Role of the NHS*, London: Health Education Authority.

West, R., Sammons, P. and West, A. (1993) 'Effects of a traffic club on road safety knowledge and self-reported behaviour of young children and their parents', *Accident Analysis and Prevention* 25: 609–18.

Young, D. S. and Lee, D. N. (1987) 'Training children in road crossing skills using a roadside simulation', *Accident Analysis and Prevention* 19: 327–41.

Chapter 8

Child sexual abuse: myth and reality

Bill Gillham

The mid-1990s provides a standpoint for placing child sexual abuse in perspective. It has presumably always been with us but, in the UK at least, fifteen years ago the topic had no place in public awareness. The earliest of the new wave of US studies (e.g. Finkelhor, 1979) were known to a few specialist professionals, yet social work departments typically did not list sexual abuse as a separate (or significant) category in their classification of child abuse cases; and it was well into the 1980s before the classification was at all widely used (e.g. Wild, 1986).

There followed a period of popular and professional over-reaction, often as ill-informed as it was sincere. Popular writers (e.g. Search, 1988) wrote about an 'epidemic' of child sexual abuse. The dangers of this style of reaction became apparent through the so-called Cleveland Inquiry (DHSS, 1988) chaired by Mrs Butler-Sloss, QC, whose report is a model of integrity and good sense. The influence of that report has been profound because it serves as a cautionary tale without diminishing the importance of tackling a major social evil: one that presents distinctive problems in identification and prevention. The report is required reading for anyone with a serious professional interest in the topic; and it is, in its under-stated way, an extremely readable document.

DEFINING CHILD SEXUAL ABUSE

Kelly *et al.* (1991) set out the importance of this fundamental question as follows:

> How researchers define aspects of social reality has a major impact on their 'findings', and these 'findings' influence both public perception and social policy. The influence of definitions, however, is seldom made clear to non-researchers, and is often perceived as irrelevant and 'technical'. This frequently results in misunderstandings and misre-presentations which have potentially far reaching consequences. The conflation of incidence and prevalence figures, for example, produces

estimates in the media (which have also been used in practitioner training) that 1 in 4 or 1 in 10 (depending on the study used) children are currently being abused, as opposed to the correct interpretation that this proportion of children will experience some form of abuse before they are 16–18. Similarly where it is unclear what is included within the term 'sexual abuse in childhood' prevalence figures are frequently interpreted as referring to ongoing abuse, usually in a familial context. (p. 14)

There is no shortage of definitions. Fraser (1981) suggests: 'the exploit-ation of a child for the sexual gratification of an adult' (p. 58). No doubt we would all agree with that, but it is nowhere near precise enough. What is a child? (and what is an adult?). And what is meant by 'sexual gratification'?

The age of 'consent' – the notion that before this age children cannot be held to consent to sexual activity – provides a legal framework. In English law this relates to sexual intercourse, either heterosexual, i.e. by a man over 16 with a girl under 16, or homosexual, by a man over 18 with a male under 18. Note that these formulations exclude female sexual abusers.

The legal age of consent has varied over time and, indeed, within one country. In the US the age of consent varies from one state to another, the range being 12 to 18 years, although the usual age is 16. This age of consent has been established in English law only since 1885; before that it was 13 (Vinnika, 1989). And it should be noted that sexual intercourse with a girl under 13 remains a separate offence from intercourse with a girl over 13 but under 16.

The raising of the age of consent in Victorian England was a response to social concern about the large number of child prostitutes, there being tens of thousands of these in London alone (Pinchbeck and Hewitt, 1973). This legislation was part of a late response to the need to protect children and is outlined in the chapter on physical abuse. The special, protected status of childhood which we now take for granted is, in fact, a compara-tively recent phenomenon, the earliest manifestations being not more than two hundred years old (Ariès, 1962).

The criteria for defining 'childhood' victims in sexual abuse research range from those in the pre-puberty category (e.g. Fritz *et al.*, 1981) to those under 18 (e.g. Wyatt, 1985). This parallels variations in the legal age of consent.

How does one define an abuse? Baker and Duncan (1985), as part of a UK prevalence study employed the following definition:

A child (anyone under 16 years) is sexually abused when another person, who is sexually mature, involves the child in any activity which the other person expects to lead to their sexual arousal. (p. 458)

But sexual maturity typically occurs before the age of 16 and approximately a fifth of all sexual offences (including rape) in England and Wales are committed by those who are legally children (Home Office, 1994).

The concepts of 'consent' and 'abuse' vary according to the age-difference between those involved. Sexual activity between post-pubertal but 'under age' children is so common as to be general (Ingham, 1994). Without mutual consent this becomes 'peer abuse' but the distinction is not easy to make. However, a 15-year-old who engaged in sexual activity with a 5-year-old would unquestionably be regarded as an abuser. Hence, the age-gap is an important factor in an operational definition of abuse.

One widely used definition is that of the influential American researcher, David Finkelhor of the University of New Hampshire, as follows:

- a sexual encounter between a child of 12 and under with a person of 19 or over;
- where the child is under 12 and the other person under 19 but at least 5 years older;
- where a child/adolescent is 13 to 16 years and the other person is at least 10 years older.

(Finkelhor, 1979)

Note that this excludes peer sexual abuse. Although less easy to define (it is necessarily more subjective), any debate as to whether peer abuse constitutes child sexual abuse is playing with words: abuse in any context has to be recognised and dealt with.

When is something sexual? As seducers well know there is a subtle gradient here. It is most unambiguous when actual contact is involved and hence the focus of preventative work on the touch continuum (e.g. Gillham, 1995). The complicating factor is that normal adult care of children may well involve touching the genitals or other 'private' parts of the body. A distinction is usually made between 'contact' and 'non-contact' forms of abuse. Contact abuse ranges from fondling and sexual kissing to vaginal and anal intercourse and oral–genital sex. Non-contact sex involves exhibitionism, talking about things in an erotic fashion, or showing the child pornographic material.

Not that it is quite so simple. For example, an adult who allows a child to see him or her naked may or may not be behaving with sexual intent. Those who have read (and even those who have not!) Eric Berne's *Games People Play* (1964) will be alert to what goes on in interpersonal 'transactions'.

Violence is not usually a part of child sexual abuse (Finkelhor *et al.*, 1990), nor is there often overt coercion. Seduction and enticement are the main means for the adult to achieve control. Child molesters' accounts of how they set about identifying and involving their victims are disturbing in the sophisticated calculation of their techniques (Budin and Johnson, 1989).

Child sexual abuse differs from physical abuse in a number of respects which will be considered later. A key distinction (and contrary to popular assumption) is that whereas physical abuse occurs mainly within the immediate family, most sexual abuse occurs outside it.

To return to the import of the quotation from Kelly *et al.* above, the issue of how much sexual abuse takes place *is to a large extent a function of definition*. Over-extensive definitions make the problem appear unmanageable and divert attention away from those children most at risk from the more serious forms of abuse. As we shall see in the section on incidence and prevalence that follows, most children's experience of 'sexual abuse' in their entire lifetime is of a single event of a relatively minor character.

INCIDENCE AND PREVALENCE

These two terms mean quite different things although they are often used interchangeably. *Prevalence* studies attempt to estimate the proportion of a population that has been sexually abused during childhood; while *incidence* studies seek to estimate the number of new cases occurring in a given period of time, usually a year. In practice, incidence studies are of reported cases; of necessity these are biased and this bias is amplified when whole-population estimates are derived from them. Both approaches can misrepresent (or appear to misrepresent) the scale of the problem.

Prevalence studies involve asking an adult (usually a young adult) population, by questionnaire or interview, whether they experienced sexual abuse in childhood. These studies yield fairly high rates for abuse, averaging around 30 per cent for girls and 15 per cent for boys (Gillham, 1991: 8) but the figures are typically inflated in two ways:

- all incidents including the relatively minor are usually counted;
- the figures reflect a childhood lifetime perspective, i.e. around ten years of reliable recall – all problems can appear large if we aggregate over a long period of time.

If we exclude the less serious (and often minor) incidents and consider that the figures must then be divided by approximately ten (years), then the current scale of the problem is much less than might appear from headlines proclaiming that x per cent of girls, etc. are abused.

There is one other bias in prevalence studies and it is this: that many investigations focus only on populations of women, e.g. the recent New Zealand study by Anderson *et al.* (1993). This exclusion of male victims carries its own kind of cultural message, is part of the social construction of sexual abuse – a theme we shall return to.

Incidence studies are more systematically biased. An aggregate analysis of studies up to 1990 (Gillham, 1991: 7–22) provides the basis for what follows. Subsequent studies have not altered the picture. Incidence data are given on the left; prevalence data on the right.

1 *Ratio of girls to boys*   *Incidence*   *Prevalence*
                              Approximately 7:1   Approximately 2:1

Comment: Some incidence studies report negligible incidence rates for boys (e.g. James *et al.* (1978) which reports *none*). As research has proceeded relatively more abuse of boys has become apparent (e.g. Spencer and Dunklee, 1986).

2 *Experience of contact abuse*   *Incidence*   *Prevalence*
                                   Mainly girls   Mainly boys

Comment: The most representative UK prevalence study (Baker and Duncan, 1985: 461) reported boys experiencing *more* contact abuse than girls. Goldman and Goldman (1988: 99), in an Australian prevalence study, reported that boys were three times as likely to experience the most serious forms of abuse. Non-contact abuse, e.g. by exhibitionists, is almost entirely directed at girls; Finkelhor (1979: 62) in a prevalence study reported that 20 per cent of the female sample's experiences were of this type. However, *incestuous* abuse occurs more often to girls (see below).

3 *Proportion of female abusers*   *Incidence*   *Prevalence*
                                    Less than 3 per cent   About 6 per cent of
                                                            abuse of girls and 56
                                                            per cent of abuse of boys

Comment: The higher figures for female abuse of boys come from US studies of college students (e.g. Fromuth and Burkhart, 1987).

4 *Abuse by strangers*   *Incidence*   *Prevalence*
                          About 17 per cent   About 42 per cent

Comment: This is almost the inverse of what follows.

5 *Intrafamilial abuse*   *Incidence*   *Prevalence*
                           About 45 per cent   About 23 per cent

Comment: This consistent finding is important because the popular and often the professional conception is that 'incest is the most common form of sexual abuse' (Risin and MacNamara, 1989: 179, para. 1; see also Armstrong's 1978 book entitled *Kiss Daddy Goodnight*). This kind of emphasis often has strong feminist motives, e.g. Driver (1989). Russell (1983) in one of the best executed prevalence studies of the sexual abuse of women found that the most serious forms of abuse were more than twice as likely to occur *outside* the family. It is, however, the case that girls are more likely to be abused by relatives than boys. Finkelhor (1979) gives a figure of 43 per cent of reported incidents for girls as against 17 per cent for boys. Goldman and Goldman (1988) giving very similar figures also report a rate of 0.5 per cent for girls experiencing sexual intercourse with a blood relative, twice the rate for boys. Using the same definition Baker and Duncan (1985) report a prevalence rate of 0.25 per cent. In Nash and West's (1985) study (questionnaire data) three out of 315 women reported sexual contact with their biological father (including one case of sexual intercourse and another of attempted intercourse); five women reported sexual contact with a stepfather/father figure; and three more reported sexual contact with a brother (including one case of intercourse). In the larger study of 1,244 young people by Kelly *et al.* (1991) eight women and one man reported sexual intercourse with a relative, an overall rate of 0.64 per cent. The prevalence of 'classic' incest at around one woman in 200 and one man in 500 is lower than one might expect from reading some of the literature, but it does, of course, represent the most severe form of abuse with the most severe psychological consequences (Green, 1993).

6 *Social class*	*Incidence*	*Prevalence*
	Mainly lower (i.e. manual) socioeconomic groups	Equally (pro-rata) distributed across all social classes

Comment: Incidence studies (i.e. of cases reported to medical and social work agencies) do not always report the socioeconomic composition of the referred cases; this is especially true of medical reports. Social work agencies do this more often (e.g. Russell and Trainor, 1984; Creighton, 1992). The latter, NSPCC longitudinal study, is the major source of data in the UK. However, Social Work Departments work almost exclusively with and for the socially disadvantaged sections of the community. Because sexual abuse is less 'visible' than physical abuse (which is largely defined by visible evidence of injury) it tends to be detected mainly in those families which come under scrutiny for other reasons. This 'fortuitous' factor was particularly evident in the cases involved in the Cleveland Inquiry, cited above. And within Social Work Departments some social workers are more expert (or more enthusiastic) in the detection of sexual abuse. The scope for bias is, therefore, very great: in those cases referred in the first instance; and in those detected because of specialist interest or concern.

This summary account of the very different picture one gets according to the method of data collection employed goes a long way to explaining why different people (including professionals and researchers) have a different picture of child sexual abuse. However, it is *not* the 'methodological quagmire' described by Dempster and Roberts (1991). What it does is to emphasise the importance of asking these questions of any study:

- is it an incidence or prevalence study?
- how is sexual abuse defined?
- how representative is the population studied?
- how was the data obtained?

PREVALENCE STUDIES IN THE UK

Because prevalence studies are more representative than incidence studies we shall concentrate on those in our attempt to analyse the problem more closely. There are three main UK studies: those of Baker and Duncan, 1985; Nash and West, 1985; and Kelly *et al.*, 1991. Summary statistics are given in Table 8.1; each study will be considered in turn because each has something unique to offer. Firstly some differences in method between the studies.

There are three main ways of getting a population sample: by random or *probability* sampling; by *quota* sampling; and by so-called *convenience* sampling. In a probability sample each member of the population from which it is drawn has an equal chance of being selected. It is therefore truly representative. There are, however, two drawbacks:

- it is expensive and troublesome to do;
- many of the randomly selected individuals may (and usually do) decline to cooperate.

For these reasons surveys usually take a quota sample: researchers are given a nationally representative quota (e.g. by age, social class and gender) and approach individuals who fit the requirements and agree to cooperate. Such a group is representative in fitting the quota requirements but unrepresentative in that they have all agreed to take part. This sampling method came adrift in the opinion polls in the 1992 UK general election. People who agree to be interviewed are apparently more likely to be left-wing (Curtice, 1994).

A convenience sample is a euphemism for a group the researcher can access fairly easily: student groups are commonly used for this reason. Looking at Table 8.1 below we see that two of the studies employed convenience samples. There is no way of knowing how representative these groups are, though the study by Kelly *et al.* comes close to a quota sample in social class terms.

This does not mean that the Baker and Duncan study is superior. Here the main weakness is that the investigation was 'piggy-backed' on a MORI general household survey. Individuals were asked a single question as to whether they had ever experienced any form of sexual abuse: if they said 'yes' further questions were asked. The context of the interview was probably not one to encourage disclosure on such a sensitive matter. It remains, however, the largest and most representative study to date.

Table 8.1 Summary statistics of three UK prevalence studies of child sexual abuse

Study	Sample	Data collection	Definition	Age of victim	% reporting abuse	% reporting familial abuse	Sex of abuser
Baker and Duncan (1985)	Quota sample (Male and female) N = 2019	Interview	Contact and non-contact	Under 16	F = 12 M = 8	1.4	'Vast majority' male
Nash and West (1985)	Convenience sample (i) 94 F on GP list (ii) 50 F college students (part sample)	Questionnaire and interview	Contact and non-contact	Under 16	(i) 42 (ii) 54	(i) 7.6 (ii) 9.2	99% male
Kelly *et al.* (1991)	Convenience sample N = 1244 Students in FE colleges 62% F 38% M	Questionnaire	Contact and non-contact	Under 18 Under 16	F = 59 M = 27 F = 36 M = 19	F = 5.9 M = 1.35	5% female (also 15% by age-peers)

Not all of the three studies present the same kind of data. Two findings from the Baker and Duncan study are worthy of particular note, as follows.

Age of first experience of sexual abuse

Baker and Duncan (p. 459) report an average of 12.03 years for boys and 10.74 years for girls. These ages are slightly higher than in the US studies by Finkelhor (1979: 60; 1984: 73) and the Australian study by Goldman and Goldman (1988: 98). What all the studies do is challenge the very general assumption that it is the development of secondary sexual characteristics which renders girls particularly vulnerable to abuse. Clearly *pre-pubertal* girls are most at risk. The finding that boys are at risk of abuse at an older age is consistent across all published prevalence studies.

Social class and sexual abuse

Although cases of sexual abuse referred to or detected by Social Work Departments are overwhelmingly from the manual social classes (in the UK C2, D and E), (Creighton, 1992), prevalence studies show no such pattern. One of the most interesting findings in the Baker and Duncan study is that there were 'no significant differences between the abused, non-abused and refused-to-answer groups with regard to social class' (p. 459). Reviewing the main US studies Finkelhor (1987) comments that they 'are fairly uniform in failing to find differences in rates according to social class or racial subdivision' (p. 234).

It follows that middle-class sexually abused children are less likely to be detected and protected and this may have particular consequences for them. It is worth noting here that eating disorders (anorexia nervosa and bulimia) are more common amongst middle-class than working-class young women and that sexual abuse appears to be one of the contributory causes in at least some cases (Herzog *et al.*, 1993).

But how could these cases remain hidden? The answer is: quite easily, the problem being the 'low visibility' and, in the past, the low credibility of sexual abuse. Middle-class families are both more private and less suspected than their socially disadvantaged counterparts. A special problem in sexual abuse is the evidence factor (Gillham, 1992). Well-meaning attempts at intervention can easily fail at this level.

SEXUAL ABUSE AND THE PROBLEM OF EVIDENCE

In the UK the popular 'discovery' of sexual abuse is a phenomenon of the past decade. There followed a period of over-reaction focused in the UK in the much-publicised Cleveland Inquiry (DHSS, 1988) and, subsequently, a cautionary backlash (Hobbs and Wynne, 1990: 424).

The Cleveland Inquiry brought into sharp focus the problem of evidence in determining that child sexual abuse had occurred. Of particular contention was the use of a test of reflex anal dilatation as evidence of buggery, but all kinds of evidence were reviewed and the means used for collating and interpreting them.

What the report revealed was a situation where various professionals of undoubted integrity held strong views which did not pay sufficient regard to scientific standards of medical and psychological evidence. As the Report makes clear, the paediatricians at the centre of the controversy were dedicated to the care and welfare of children. One can well understand the impact of the 1986 conference presentation by Dr Wynne on Dr Higgs (her first diagnosis of sexual abuse based on an anal examination came some four weeks later). Doctors Hobbs and Wynne's paper published in *The Lancet* in the same year (Hobbs and Wynne, 1986) describing cases of buggery involving very young children cannot be read without feelings of anger.

Previous to the Cleveland Inquiry the failures of child abuse identification procedures had centred on 'false negatives', as in the case of Maria Colwell, where there was a failure to ascertain the level of risk to which the child was exposed. *False positives*, that is where non-accidental injury was wrongly diagnosed or children were incorrectly judged to be at risk, have always been given much less attention, despite the distress they have undoubtedly caused, presumably because of professional justification on the 'better safe than sorry' principle.

The Cleveland Inquiry highlighted the consequences of false positives in identifying children as sexually abused with the associated trauma for both the children and their parents. Let it be affirmed, however, that a significant number of children were correctly diagnosed (see Part One, Chapter One of the Butler-Sloss Report). What was disturbing was Dr Higgs' difficulty in accepting that *any* of her diagnoses could have been wrong (DHSS, 1988: 142). It now seems likely that there were more false positives than true positives. Much of the problem lies in the relatively low incidence of sexual abuse in the child population, and the statistical probabilities of misdiagnoses, i.e. false positives that stem from this.

We do not yet have adequate prevalence studies of child sexual abuse in the UK. The nearest is the study, based on a quota sample of personal interviews, reported by Baker and Duncan in 1985. Of the 2019 people interviewed, 10 per cent reported at least one incident which could be considered abusive during their childhood. However, many of these were minor, e.g. exhibitionism or relatively slight physical contact. Only a small proportion of these incidents (5 per cent of the 10 per cent, i.e. 0.5 per cent over all) amounted to full sexual intercourse, boys being equally at risk as girls (Baker and Duncan, 1985: 461). Goldman and Goldman (1988) provide similar data for an Australian population (see Table 6,

p. 99) but found that 1.5 per cent of the children (again, equally boys and girls) experienced full intercourse.

Children who have been sexually abused may well show emotional and behavioural symptoms of psychological disturbance: the problem lies in the reverse inference. A large percentage, perhaps even a majority, of children are psychologically disturbed at some time in their lives (Douglas, 1989; Rutter *et al.*, 1970); the causes are multiple and the range of symptoms limited. Sink (1988: 131) emphasises that: 'with the exception of precocious and atypical sexualizing behaviors in some children, the patterns observed are not specific to abused children'.

Powell (1991) in a review of the research evidence on psychological assessment comments: 'the presence of psychological or behavioural problems should never be regarded as evidence that abuse has occurred in a particular case' (p. 78). Powell's paper is recommended as an authoritative and up to date summary, extensively referenced. A final quotation from that paper takes us a stage further: 'there is no accurate quantitative method by which psychologists can evaluate evidence of sexual abuse, *and any diagnosis where there has been no confession or disclosure is based solely on inference*' (p. 77) (emphasis added).

Facilitating disclosure by very young children without contaminating their evidence (because such it is to a psychologist as much as to a lawyer) is a skill of high order. The problem in communication is the enormous gap in knowledge and understanding between the child and the adult. DeYoung (1987) puts this very well: 'The act of sexual abuse is a complex behavior that involves not only the act *per se* but an intricate network of corresponding motives, feelings, attitudes, perceptions, and assumptions that adults must understand in order to define and assess the act, but which the young child is largely unable to comprehend or communicate' (p. 219).

Thus children are likely not to 'make sense' of what happened in adult terms; for the same reason they may miss out what, to an adult, might seem important (e.g. contextual) details. Young children tend to recall less detail, but what they say in *free recall* is as accurate as an adult account (Raskin and Yuille, 1989). *Errors* of detail seem to be the consequence of leading or suggestive questioning by adults (Yuille, 1988).

But do children never lie about sexual abuse? It is commonly asserted that they do so only rarely (e.g. Kidscape (undated); DeJong 1985: 512). Yuille (1988) in a review of American studies reported that fewer than 10 per cent of allegations were false: a small proportion, but one warranting the description 'uncommon' rather than 'rare'. Raskin and Yuille (1989) comment that fictitious accounts are typically made in the context of divorce, custody and visitation disputes.

How are false allegations characterised? In her review Powell (1991: 81) concludes that there are three main indicators:

- the use of adult terminology and expressions;
- marked contradiction and variation of the central details of the story across time;
- accounts which are more 'verbal' than 'visual'.

This last point is an important one. In a true allegation there may be gaps in the child's account, but the details given suggest something that has been *witnessed* rather than verbally rehearsed.

The problem of helping young children to translate their witness experience into an adequate form of words is a considerable one and sometimes impossible for intellectual and linguistic reasons as much as emotional and social immaturity. The use of anatomically detailed dolls, i.e. with realistic genitals, anal orifice, etc. is increasing in this country and widespread in the US. It is, however, quite clear that they should be seen as an aid to communication rather than as a means of diagnosing sexual abuse. A child who involves the dolls in explicit sexual activity may be reflecting abusive experiences but it may also indicate that he or she has observed adults in sexual activity within the family situation – unsurprising in view of the conditions in which some families have to live.

The most secure evidence appears to be medical diagnosis soon after the offences (less than 72 hours: Finkel, 1989: 1145) and the child's facilitated but unenhanced disclosure. One problem is that disclosure is often much delayed. For example, in a study of 311 *severe* cases of abuse (Rimsza and Niggeman, 1982) 55 per cent of the children delayed reporting for longer than 72 hours and 30 per cent only reported after multiple episodes.

A related problem is that children often find the adult reaction to disclosure even more traumatic than the abuse itself (e.g. Gagnon, 1965: 184). Adult women interviewed by Nash and West (1985) about their disclosure in childhood of experiences of sexual abuse were very critical of their treatment by social workers, police and doctors (p. 63). Even where the disclosure is more sympathetically received it is likely to be made to adults without experience or training in handling the child's desire to communicate. And even if what the child says is adequately recorded, the questions put *to* the child may not be, so that the primary source of evidence soon becomes overlaid with unknown influences.

A concern about the quality of evidence may seem an excessively 'legalistic' or 'scientific' preoccupation. A well-intentioned conviction that abuse has occurred when the evidence has not been properly evaluated can result in psychological damage for everyone concerned. Even when abuse *has* occurred the professional response may be disturbing and harmful. The consequences of false accusation are disastrous in human terms. Dennis Howitt's (1992) book *Child Abuse Errors* describes many such cases.

CONCLUSION

This chapter has highlighted the difficulties of gaining an accurate picture of the scale and character of child sexual abuse, and the importance of sifting the research evidence so that 'common knowledge', which so badly misrepresents the reality, is brought into line with the evidence.

REFERENCES

Anderson, J., Martin, J., Mullen, P., Romans, S. and Herbison, P. (1993) 'Prevalence of childhood sexual abuse experiences in a community sample of women', *Journal of the American Academy of Child and Adolescent Psychiatry* 32, 5: 911–19.

Ariès, P. (1962) *Centuries of Childhood*, London: Jonathan Cape.

Armstrong, L. (1978) *Kiss Daddy Goodnight*, New York: Hawthorn.

Baker, A.W. and Duncan, S.P. (1985) 'Child sexual abuse: a study of prevalence in Great Britain', *Child Abuse and Neglect* 9, 4: 457–67.

Berne, E. (1964) *Games People Play*, Harmondsworth: Penguin Books.

Budin, L.E. and Johnson, C.F. (1989) 'Sex abuse prevention programs: offenders' attitudes about their efficacy', *Child Abuse and Neglect* 13, 1: 77–87.

Creighton, S.J. (1992) *Child Abuse Trends in England and Wales 1988–1990*. London: NSPCC.

Curtice, J. (1994) 'What future for the opinion poll? The lessons of the MRS inquiry', *Scottish Affairs* 10: 1–20.

DeJong, A.R. (1985) 'The medical evaluation of sexual abuse in children', *Hospital and Community Psychology* 36, 5: 509–12.

DeYoung, M. (1987) 'Disclosing sexual abuse: the impact of developmental variables', *Child Welfare* 66: 217–33.

DHSS (1988) *Report of the Inquiry into Child Abuse in Cleveland 1987*, London: HMSO.

Dempster, H.L. and Roberts, J. (1991) 'Child sexual abuse: a methodological quagmire', *Child Abuse and Neglect* 15: 593–5.

Douglas, J. (1989) *Behaviour Problems in Young Children*, London: Routledge.

Driver, E. (1989) 'Introduction', in E. Driver and A. Druisen (eds) *Child Sexual Abuse: Feminist Perspectives*, London: Macmillan.

Finkel, M.A. (1989) 'Child sexual abuse: a physician's introduction to historical and medical validation', *Journal of the American Osteopathic Association* 89, 9: 1143–9.

Finkelhor, D. (1979) *Sexually Victimized Children*, New York: Free Press.

—— (1984) *Child Sexual Abuse: New Theory and Research*, London: Collier Macmillan.

—— (1987) 'The sexual abuse of children: current research reviewed', *Psychiatric Annals* 17, 4: 233–41.

Finkelhor, D., Hotaling, G., Lewis, I.A. and Smith, C. (1990) 'Sexual abuse in a national survey of adult men and women: Prevalence, characteristics and risk factors', *Child Abuse and Neglect* 14, 1: 19–28.

Fraser, B.G. (1981) 'Sexual child abuse: the legislation and the law in the United States', in P.B. Mrazek and C.H. Kempe (eds) *Sexually Abused Children and Their Families*, New York: Pergamon.

Fritz, G.S., Stoll, K. and Wagner, N. (1981) 'A comparison of males and females who were sexually molested as children', *Journal of Sex and Marital Therapy* 7, 1: 54–9.

Fromuth, M. and Burkhart, B. (1987) 'Childhood sexual victimization among college men: definitional and methodological issues', *Violence and Victims* 2, 4: 241–53.

Gagnon, J.H. (1965) 'Female child victims of sex offences', *Social Problems* 13, 2: 176–92.

Gillham, B. (1991) *Child Sexual Abuse*, London: Cassell.

Gillham, B. (1992) 'Evidence in cases of child sexual abuse', *Journal of the Law Society of Scotland* 37, 6: 225–8.

Gillham, B. (1995) *In Touch – O.K., Not O.K.*, Glasgow: BBC2.

Goldman, R.J. and Goldman, J.D.G. (1988) 'The prevalence and nature of sexual abuse in Australia', *Australian Journal of Sex, Marriage and Family* 9, 2: 94–106.

Green, A.H. (1993) 'Child sexual abuse: immediate and long-term effects and intervention', *Journal of the American Academy of Adolescent and Child Psychiatry* 32, 5: 890–902.

Herzog, K.B., Staley, J.E., Carmody, S., Robbins, W.M. and van der Kolk, B.A. (1993) 'Child sexual abuse in anorexia nervosa and bulimia nervosa: a pilot study', *Journal of the American Academy of Child and Adolescent Psychiatry* 32, 5: 962–6.

Hobbs, C.J. and Wynne, J.M. (1986) 'Buggery in childhood – a common syndrome of child abuse', *Lancet* 2: 792–6.

—— (1990) 'The sexually abused battered child', *Archives of Disease in Childhood* 65, 4: 423–7.

Home Office (1994) *Criminal Statistics England and Wales 1993*, London: HMSO.

Howitt, D. (1992) *Child Abuse Errors*, London: Harvester Wheatsheaf.

Ingham, R. (1994) 'Some speculations on the concept of rationality', in G. Albrecht (ed.) *Advances in Medical Sociology* (Vol. IV), Greenwich, Conn.: JAI Press.

James, J., Womack, W.M. and Strauss, F. (1978) 'Physician reporting of sexual abuse of children', *Journal of the American Medical Association* 240, 11: 1145–6.

Kelly, L., Regan, L. and Burton, S. (1991) 'An exploratory study of sexual abuse in a sample of 16–21 year olds', *End of Award Report R000 23 1746*, Swindon: ESRC.

Kidscape (undated leaflet) *The Facts About Child Sexual Abuse*, London: Kidscape.

Nash, C.L. and West, D.J. (1985) 'Sexual molestation of young girls: a retrospective survey', in D.J. West (ed.) *Sexual Victimization*, Aldershot: Gower Publishing.

Pinchbeck, I. and Hewitt, M. (1973) *Children in English Society* (Vol. 2), London: Routledge and Kegan Paul.

Powell, M.B. (1991) 'Investigating and reporting child sexual abuse: review and recommendations for clinical practice', *Australian Psychologist* 26, 2: 77–83.

Raskin, D.C. and Yuille, J.C. (1989) 'Problems in evaluating interviews of children in sexual abuse cases', in S.J. Ceci, D.F. Ross and M.P. Toglia (eds) *Perspectives on Children's Testimony*, New York: Springer-Verlag.

Rimsza, M.E. and Niggeman, E.H. (1982) 'Medical evaluation of sexually abused children: a review of 311 cases', *Pediatrics* 69, 1: 8–14.

Risin, L.I. and MacNamara, J.R. (1989) 'Validation of child sexual abuse: the psychologist's role', *Journal of Clinical Psychology* 45, 1: 175–84.

Russell, A.B. and Trainor, C.M. (1984) *Trends in Child Abuse and Neglect*, Denver: American Humane Association.

Russell, D.E.H. (1983) 'The incidence and prevalence of intrafamilial and extrafamilial sexual abuse of female children', *Child Abuse and Neglect* 7: 133–46.

Rutter, M., Tizard, J. and Whitmore, K. (1970) *Education, Health and Behaviour*, London: Longman.

Search, G. (1988) *The Last Taboo: Sexual Abuse of Children*, Harmondsworth: Penguin Books.

Sink, F. (1988) 'A hierarchical model for evaluation of child sexual abuse', *American Journal of Orthopsychiatry* 58, 1: 129–35.

Spencer, M.J. and Dunklee, P. (1986) 'Sexual abuse of boys', *Pediatrics* 78, 1: 133–8.

Vinnika, S. (1989) 'Child sexual abuse and the law', in E. Driver and A. Druisen (eds) *Child Sexual Abuse: Feminist Perspectives*, London: Macmillan.

Wild, N.J. (1986) 'Sexual abuse of children in Leeds', *British Medical Journal* 292: 1113–16.

Wyatt, G.E. (1985) 'The sexual abuse of Afro-American and White American women in childhood', *Child Abuse and Neglect* 9: 507–19.

Yuille, J.C. (1988) 'The systematic assessment of children's testimony', *Canadian Psychology* 29: 247–62.

Chapter 9

The prevention of child sexual abuse

David Warden

The natural response of most adults to the sexual abuse of a child is one of anger, disgust and, most probably, an inclination to disbelief. How is it possible that anyone could act in such a way? Strong emotions do, however, create an impetus for action, and within the last decade and a half, considerable efforts have been made towards the prevention of abuse and the protection of children. Such efforts have had three general aims:

- to rehabilitate child sex offenders in the hope of preventing further abuse;
- to educate children about safety issues, such that they are better able to recognise and protect themselves from potential harm, and know what to do if they are made to feel unsafe;
- to educate parents, teachers and the wider community about safer child-rearing practices, about the detection of possible abuse, and about the myths surrounding child abuse.

This chapter will focus on the latter two educational aims. It will present a critical review of recent safety training and abuse prevention programmes, a discussion of the content of such programmes, their conceptual, ethical, administrative and presentational problems, and the extent to which evaluation has demonstrated their success. We shall also consider some of the problems faced by parents, teachers and educational authorities in guiding and protecting children in this area.

EDUCATING CHILDREN

The aims of child sexual abuse prevention programmes are (1) to improve the knowledge and awareness of children such that they can recognise and avoid situations in which abuse may occur, (2) to develop the necessary behavioural skills (e.g. assertiveness) which could assist them in dealing with unsafe situations, and (3) to encourage children to disclose previous or ongoing abuse. While these are legitimate aims it should, of course, never be assumed that such programmes in any way relieve adults of ultimate responsibility for children's safety.

What gains in children's knowledge and behaviour do safety training programmes seek to foster?

A plethora of safety training packages has appeared in the last ten to fifteen years, addressing different age groups, from pre-school to teenage, and different aspects of abuse, both physical and sexual, and employing different methods of presentation. The majority of these have been developed and used in America, but some recent British programmes include Kidscape, *Feeling Yes, Feeling No* (Educational Media International, 1985), *Better Safe Than Sorry* (Educational Media International, 1986), and *Say No, Don't Go* (Scottish Office Home and Health Department, 1992). The addresses for these teaching materials are in the References at the end of this chapter. A fuller summary of prevention programmes can be found in Mayes *et al.*, (1992).

Despite the wide variety of programmes, all address in one way or another the same basic questions, namely, what is sexual abuse? who does it? and what can you do to avoid it? The concept of sexual abuse has frequently been explained with reference to 'good' and 'bad' touching. Children are encouraged to appreciate the privacy of their bodies, and their ownership thereof, and to distinguish positive, caring and welcome touching from unwelcome attempts at physical intimacy. Programmes also attempt to give guidance on the likely source of abuse. A convenient approach to this difficult topic has sometimes been to talk about abuse in the context of 'stranger-danger', an approach given credence by public paranoia about 'stranger abductions'. However, it is now more widely recognised that a child abuser is likely to be familiar to the child, either because he or she is a family friend or relation, or because the abuser's strategy is first to become familiar with the child and to gain his or her confidence and trust. The third safety training theme addresses what a victim of potential or actual abuse can do. This may involve the training of assertiveness skills intended to give children the confidence to say no, and to be able to remove themselves from unwelcome interactions. Considerable emphasis is also given to encouraging children to report any incidents of abuse. This latter exhortation involves discussion of another difficult issue: the breaking of confidences, for abusive relationships may involve the imposition of secrecy, and feelings of guilt often attach to a decision either to tell or not to tell. What is the difference between a 'good' secret and a 'bad' secret? What secrets should you tell, why, and to whom? These are all difficult questions which require sensitive handling.

Training programmes have adopted a wide variety of presentational methods, including story-, colouring- and comic-books, videos, role-playing games, puppet shows or plays by theatre groups, and various combinations of these. Some programmes may be presented at home by the child's parents, but more commonly, they are presented at school by a teacher, a local community police officer, or by some other trained outside presenter.

The presentation of a safety training programme in schools, and its attendant difficulties, can be exemplified by Kidscape, a well-received example of the genre. Kidscape operates what it calls a concept of 'Good Sense Defence', aiming to provide 'practical ways to help children to recognise and deal with potentially dangerous situations, including the possibility of sexual abuse'. In other words, sexual abuse prevention is presented in the context of more general safety training. The training begins by teaching children general rules about what to do if they are lost, how to make an emergency telephone call, etc., before moving on to the four specific areas of potential abuse: (1) how to cope with bullies, (2) not to talk to strangers, (3) to say 'no' and to tell if someone wants them to do something which makes them feel uncomfortable, and (4) that some secrets should not be kept. The training, usually given by the class teacher, can be carried out in one block, or broken down into separate sections and incorporated into the curriculum. The different aspects of safety are dealt with using stories and/or role plays, and separate versions are provided for younger and older primary school children. Discussion is encouraged, drawing, painting and story writing can be used to expand upon and reinforce the themes, and posters and quiz sheets are provided to be completed with parents at home. In principle, such a programme can be effective in helping young children to understand potential dangers and to consider how to meet and deal with them. There are, however, problems of implementation which must be borne in mind.

The decision to introduce a safety training programme into the school curriculum will normally be made by a local education authority, and will depend upon the resources available to it. All schools in the region will then be provided with a training pack. However laudable the political decision to introduce abuse prevention programmes into schools, and however enthusiastic and well intentioned are the head teachers who espouse their use, it is the class teachers who must present them, who must find ways to talk to the children in their classrooms about the demanding topic of child sexual abuse. A moment's consideration suggests that no one would find this easy: to handle it at all, let alone to do it with sensitivity and tact, is a task of considerable proportions. Class teachers, as prospective trainers, must be given training and support, both in the presentation of the package, and in the procedures for dealing with any problems that may arise such as, most obviously, the disclosure of, or suspected cases of abuse. Most local education authorities do now have guidelines and procedures for dealing with suspected abuse. However, experience suggests that individual teacher training and support services are variable, and subject to resource allocation. In consequence, teachers, already burdened with a heavy teaching and administrative load, find that they are asked to take on not only an additional teaching commitment, but also one that they may feel will cause them embarrassment and possibly distress. Without clear support, this can only have negative consequences for the enthusiasm, thoroughness and regularity with which classroom sessions are tackled.

How effective are safety training programmes?

The introduction of abuse prevention education into the lives of young children has not always been matched by an evaluation of its effect upon the safety and well-being of its recipients. How much knowledge and awareness do children gain from safety training programmes, how stable is such learning, and what behavioural consequences ensue? Does greater knowledge and awareness cause children to be safer? Does safety training result in children being more suspicious, nervous or alienated in their dealings with adults?

Several methodological, conceptual and ethical difficulties arise when attempts are made to evaluate the effects of safety training. For example, if success is to be measured in terms of greater safety, how can we quantify what has not happened, i.e. what has been prevented, when statistics on the incidence of abuse remain uncertain? Again, while we may wish to know whether a trained child will behave more safely than an untrained child in a dangerous situation, we can hardly place children in dangerous situations to find out. A further problem is that the essence of evaluation is comparative, to determine which education programme works best? But prevention programmes differ in so many respects – Conte *et al.* (1986) suggest seven dimensions of variability – that comparison between them is not easy. There is also the problem of evaluating programme effectiveness with different age groups. While interviews, or paper and pencil tasks, or even role plays may be feasible with older primary school children, preschool and early primary school children cannot participate so easily in such evaluation attempts. It is also the case that, in many of the early evaluations, the absence of a control group and the failure to conduct a long term follow-up assessment left the question of effectiveness unanswered. Nonetheless, there have been a number of recent evaluations which allow some constructive conclusions to be drawn (Mayes *et al.*, 1990; Hazzard *et al.*, 1991; Finkelhor and Strapko, 1992; Berrick and Barth, 1992).

For the ethical reasons mentioned above, most, though not all, evaluation studies have assessed gains in children's *knowledge* rather than changes in their *behaviour*. The general finding has been that children who participate in abuse prevention programmes, even for a relatively short period of time, do demonstrate an increased awareness of safety matters and prevention skills, at least when asked to say what they would do in potentially dangerous situations. Indeed, in a recent evaluation of the Kidscape programme, Mayes *et al.* (1990) found that, for the un-trained control children in the evaluation sample, mere participation in the assessment procedures seemed to increase their safety awareness. Another feature of this investigation was the better safety awareness manifested prior to training by children in schools which volunteered to adopt the safety training programme, compared to children in schools which did not; the implication here is that the ethos of volunteering schools already encourages safety awareness. Evaluations also suggest that knowledge gains and retention tend to be a function of age, being least with preschool children and greatest with older primary children (see, for example, Tutty, 1992). Given the vulnerability of younger child-ren to abuse, this is a worrying finding, serving to emphasise once more that the ultimate responsibility for child protection rests with adults. It has further emerged that some safety concepts are easier to learn than others (see next section); that there are considerable individual differ-ences between same-aged children in their safety awareness; and that interactive learning, e.g. role play, is a more effective method of achieving knowledge gains than passive exposure to safety messages, e.g. stories and videos. A fairly consistent finding has been that gains in knowledge do decay over longer time periods, a clear reminder that training must be a continuing part of the curriculum, rather than the one-off event it frequently is.

Evaluations of the effect of training on children's subsequent behav-iour have focused on the child's level of assertiveness and ability to say no in role play situations, or, occasionally, on their responses to simulated approaches by an adult, for example, in the school corridor. The evidence suggests some improvement in children's prevention skills in these limited contexts (e.g. Fryer *et al.*, 1987), although, as Finkelhor and Strapko (1992) note, 'the acquisition of new behaviors is less reliable and less universal than the acquisition of ideas'. It must remain doubtful whether the skills demonstrated in studies employing stranger simulation tech-niques would generalise to an emotionally charged interaction between a child and a (commonly) familiar adult abuser. The other plausible be-havioural measure of the effectiveness of training would be a reduction over time in the incidence of reported cases of abuse. However, research data directly linking abuse statistics with the use of safety training pro-grammes are not currently available. Indeed, while the reporting of abuse remains such an uncertain and haphazard procedure, assessments which relied upon changes in statistics would have to be viewed with caution. For example, it has been noted that safety training can increase the likelihood that abused children will disclose the abuse, and so, in the short term, abuse statistics may rise.

Parents and teachers frequently voice concern that participation in abuse prevention programmes in general, and in behavioural simulations or role plays in particular may frighten children, desensitise them to interactions with adults, or make them view all touching in a negative light. Existing evidence (Binder *et al.*, 1987; Wurtele and Miller-Perrin, 1987) has suggested that not only were there no side effects associated with participation in training (as judged by children, parents and teachers), but that in fact it made children feel safer, and encouraged communication on the subject between parents and their children. However, the uncertainties remain, and have been argued most recently by Melton (1992).

Children's conceptual difficulties in acquiring safety concepts

Recent research evaluating the success of safety training programmes has noted that some prevention concepts are harder to learn than others (Mayes *et al.*, 1990; Finkelhor and Strapko, 1992). What must be borne in mind is that young children's thinking tends to be concrete and context bound, that they seek 'black and white' rules, and find difficulty with exceptions and qualifications. They will therefore have problems (1) in acquiring concepts which are ambiguous, whose definitions are not clear and literal, and (2) in generalising what they have learned to different contexts. Unfortunately, many safety concepts are quite abstract and ambiguous, and adults, let alone children, find clear definition to be a problem.

For example, central to almost all sexual abuse prevention programmes is the touch continuum, and the attempt to teach children the difference between good and bad, safe and unsafe touching. However, programme evaluations frequently cite lack of success in children's acquisition or retention of such a distinction. Berrick and Barth (1992) found that, after training, a significant number of six-year-olds indicated that 'touching was intrinsically bad, and should always be reported', which would seem to reflect the black-and-white nature of their thinking. The ability to make good/bad distinctions rests upon children's attribution skills (De Young, 1988) and for a young child, such judgements are more often determined by the perceived manner or by the consequences of an action rather than by its intent. Thus an act with malevolent intent which is carried out with gentleness may be interpreted positively. A fundamental problem here is that abuse usually starts not with touching but with the building up of a trusting relationship. Abusive touching may subsequently occur in confusing situations where gentle contact is accompanied by threats and the imposition of secrecy, or where intrusive sexual contact is accompanied by expressions of love. This inconsistency of physical effect and interpersonal affect is clearly going to be problematic for any attempts to teach children to identify what is acceptable touching. As Kraizer (1986) has put it – 'children are unable to reconcile "bad" touch occurring with "good" people, that is, people they love'. Rather than teaching children about touching by focusing upon their own feelings and their resulting affective state, an alternative approach which has had some success with five- and six-year-olds (Wurtele, 1987) is to place a more concrete emphasis on the protection of private parts of the body.

Conceptual difficulty also surrounds the identity of 'a stranger' and of 'stranger-danger'. Many if not all training programmes, and much informal teaching warns children to be wary of strangers, not to accept gifts, lifts or friendly overtures from them. But who are these 'strangers'? In asking children to recognise and beware of people they don't know, we are presenting a paradoxical injunction, whose interpretation is a challenge even for adults. How can children recognise someone they don't know? This dilemma was perfectly expressed by one five-year-old boy who had been given the stranger-danger message in school that day. Walking home from school with his mother, he pointed to a man on the other side of the street, and said, 'Mum, did you know that man might be a stranger?' As for the 'danger' such strangers present to the child, it has already been noted that abusers, if they are not family friends or relations, will usually adopt the stratagem of becoming familiar with a child before embarking on any abusive interactions; thus the danger (the abusive intention), camouflaged by a friendly approach, will be difficult to recognise. To compound children's dilemma further, their socialisation, which lays considerable emphasis upon the need to be obliging and obedient to adults, will conflict with the injunction to ignore stranger approaches. These dilemmas were exemplified in a recent study of children's awareness of stranger-danger (Mayes et al., 1993), in which children, aged six to ten years, were shown video sequences of individual male adults making ostensibly innocuous approaches to a child in the street, the park, the school or the home. The adult was portrayed either as very familiar to the child, as known but not familiar, or as a stranger; and the adult's approach took the form of a request, an offer or a demand. The subjects in the study were asked what the child in the video should do and why? While all age groups did show an ability to give discriminating responses, both in terms of the different types of approach, and of the familiarity of the adult, even the oldest children showed a worrying tendency to propose compliant responses to the approaches by strangers.

Children also have difficulty with the concept of secrecy, whose imposition is a feature of abusive relationships, and which is addressed by many safety training programmes. The defining feature of a secret, according to Bok (1982), is that it involves intentional hiding or concealment, and an awareness of differential knowledge – 'I know something you don't know'. Early Piagetian views that children up to the age of seven

are unaware of different knowledge states have been considerably modified by recent research within the 'theory of mind' framework (Whiten,
1991). It is now accepted, for example, that four-year-olds can create false
beliefs and identify deceitful intentions. The practice and awareness of
deception develops quite early from games of pretence and teasing. From
the complicity of pretence, in which both sender and receiver are party
to the deception, via teasing, in which complicity is playfully and
temporarily withheld by the sender, children graduate to the duplicity
of keeping secrets and telling lies, where the deceiver deliberately hides
the deception.

Pipe and Goodman (1991) point out that it is the existence of a social
contract between two people which distinguishes keeping a secret from
telling a lie. Such a contract encompasses not only the content of the
secret, but also the relationship between the imposer of the secret and the
imposee; an awareness of the motivations for, and consequences of a
decision to keep or divulge the secret; and the personal significance of all
of these factors for the participants. Safety training attempts to distinguish between good and bad secrets, and encourages children to feel free
to divulge unwanted, imposed secrets. However, children's capacity to
make such a distinction is uncertain, and the conflict engendered by the
breaking of the social contract must place great stress upon a child. Recent
research (Mayes *et al.*, 1990) indicated that young children view secrets
generally in a positive and undiscriminating manner, enjoying the sharing of
privileged information. Similarly, Plummer (1984), in a post-test evaluation of a training programme, found that 20 per cent of ten-year-olds
thought that promises should never be broken.

Exploring this further, using a variety of different kinds of secrets (e.g.
personally upsetting information, antisocial acts, foolish mistakes, happy
surprises), Warden *et al.* (in preparation) find that six- to ten-year-old
children do demonstrate an awareness that some secrets are more important to keep than others. However, when asked how they would feel about
their decision to keep or divulge a secret, those children who had decided
that the secret should be told invariably reported that they would feel
bad, this response increasing with age. Younger children who decided
not to divulge the secret were evenly divided between feeling good and
bad, but, surprisingly, the majority of older children again reported that
they would feel bad – about *not* telling. Clearly the social pressures
involved in any secrecy contract are considerable, and the more children
become aware of the motives of and consequences for the other parties in
the contract, the greater their dilemma.

Conclusions

The onset of public concern about child sexual abuse has encouraged educational authorities to introduce safety training into the school curriculum. Despite the associated difficulties, evaluations generally support such interventions. In the main, and within the limits of role-plays or interview assessments, children's safety awareness improves, teacher–child communication is enhanced, and there is little evidence of detrimental effects such as increased anxiety or desensitisation. To the extent that both training and evaluation studies require children to respond to hypothetical situations, it may be argued that these studies underestimate children's sense of personal safety in their own lives; by the same token, however, their safety awareness regarding hypothetical situations may overestimate their ability to act upon such knowledge when the need arises.

The safety message is not a clear and simple one, and we cannot expect children to understand it fully, or to assume responsibility for their own protection. The hardest concepts for children to understand are, of course, the ones that are also hardest, or most distressing to teach; for example, that bad things can be done by 'good', or friendly, or familiar people; that these 'bad things' involve touching and secrecy, both of which also have strong positive connotations; and that social rules, about politeness, obedience and respect, sometimes need to be broken. It is both difficult and regrettable to temper young children's natural and developing sociability with caution. However, simple and understandable general rules, such as 'if you don't like what someone says or does, or asks you to do, say "no" and tell someone else about it immediately', or 'if you don't like having a secret, it probably shouldn't be a secret, so find someone to tell', and even more specific warnings, such as 'people shouldn't put their hands in your pants', all provide useful guidance upon which children can act.

EDUCATING ADULTS

If it is not sufficient just to educate children, what can be done to help adults, especially parents and teachers, to get involved in protecting children from abuse?

The first task of education must be to combat the two related problems of ignorance and denial. Surveys of adult knowledge about sexual abuse tend to reveal many misconceptions and misunderstandings – about the probability of risk, the nature of abusers and of their victims. Much misinformation concerning abuse is encouraged by the media, but such ignorance is really the consequence of denial, of the unwillingness of adults, of parents, professionals and the public at large, to face up to the reality of all the kinds of ill-treatment, including sexual abuse, which are perpetrated against children. Given a general cultural reticence regarding the discussion of normal sexual matters, it is hardly surprising that adults find the topic of child sexual abuse extremely hard to address, even with each other, let alone with children. Constructive discussion of abusive behaviour will inevitably be avoided until discussion of mundane sexual matters can be achieved openly and comfortably (by adults). Further-more, children will more easily grasp the abnormality of sexual abuse once they have achieved some understanding of normal sexual behaviour.

Parents are in a uniquely important position in this regard. As Finkelhor (1984) notes, sexual abuse can begin early in life, and parents may be the only ones in a position to help; some abuse comes from within the family, and children may more readily heed such warnings from a family member; many professionals feel that 'sexual' topics should be dealt with at home; in telling children about sexual abuse, parents are opening up channels of communication which can have lasting benefits. Wurtele *et al.* (1992) also point out that parents are likely to be more sensitive to their children's level of comprehension and knowledge of related issues, such as relationships and sex; and there is no guarantee that anyone else will talk to children about abuse if parents do not. And yet, a majority of parents are reluctant to engage in discussions about sexual abuse with their children. They may feel that their own children are not in any danger, or that they are too young, and shouldn't be frightened by such topics; or they may simply have difficulty in talking about sexual matters generally. When parents do address the threat of abuse, it is often done indirectly or obliquely, by making reference to kidnapping, strangers and other ill-defined threats. The sexual parts of the discussion are often absent.

Teachers too, while being well placed to contribute to the prevention of child abuse, often feel anxious and ill equipped to cope with such teaching, and with the personal and family traumas that abuse, its identification and disclosure can provoke. Recent surveys of teachers' knowledge about and attitudes towards abuse (Briggs, 1987; Fotheringham, 1988) revealed, amongst other things, the misconception that abuse is more likely in certain types of family, and some lingering uncertainty about the reality of abuse disclosure. While the majority of teachers expressed willingness to participate in prevention or disclosure procedures, they also expressed considerable unease about such respon-sibility, and virtual unanimity about their need for better training in detection, prevention and reaction to disclosure.

One way to advance adult education is to identify the factors which inhibit them from realising their potential as prevention educators, which differentiate educators from non-educators. Finkelhor (1984) has found that socio-economic factors such as age, occupation, education, religion were inconsequential in predicting the likelihood of parents talking about abuse with their children. What makes some parents take an active role in prevention education while others do not? In a recent study of young mothers, Macleod (1994) identified a group of educators and of non-educators and looked for general and situation-specific differences between them. At the general level, her hypothesis, that Rotter's (1982) locus of control construct might distinguish mothers who do participate in prevention education from those who do not, was not substantiated. However, working within the framework of Rogers' (1983) Protection Motivation Theory, Macleod also assessed the predictive value of more situationally specific variables such as self-efficacy ('Can I do it?'), response-efficacy ('Will it work if I do?') and response cost ('How much effort will it take?'). The relevance of such coping appraisal processes to parents' motivation to educate their children has been demonstrated by Campis *et al.* (1989). Macleod also found that mothers' perceptions about the effectiveness of prevention education (response efficacy) and, particularly, about their own effectiveness as potential educators (self-efficacy) did seem to affect their willingness to educate their children about sexual abuse.

This finding has significant practical implications for parent and teacher education, and for the marketing of prevention materials. In order for adults to participate in prevention education, they need to feel competent to do so, and to feel that their contribution will be effective. While there may sometimes be some tension between parents and teachers regarding responsibility for more academic education, this would seem to be an area where cooperation is crucial.

CONCLUSIONS

The task of developing a positive approach to abuse prevention is not easy. Prevention is hindered by inhibition, ignorance and denial. The aim must be to help all parties concerned with safety education to feel more comfortable when addressing the issue of physical intimacy, and its misuse and abuse with children. Education authorities can help teaching staff by providing both training and support. Schools can also be encouraged towards an enlightened 'whole school' policy, involving parents, acknowledging the existence of the societal problem, and wanting to make a positive contribution to its alleviation; a similar strategy is already developing towards bullying in schools. Parents, perhaps by means of open discussions in local schools, can come to a better appraisal of the dangers, of their own competence as educators, and of the sensible prevention measures they can adopt locally. While young children's understanding of many safety concepts may be limited, their awareness of safe and unsafe situations and behaviours can be enhanced by classroom and familial conversation.

REFERENCES

Berrick, J. D. and Barth, R. P. (1992) 'Child sexual abuse prevention: research review and recommendations', *Social Work Research and Abstracts* 28, 4: 6–15.

Binder, R., Dale, E. and McNeil, D. (1987) 'Evaluation of a school-based sexual abuse prevention programme: cognitive and emotional effects', *Child Abuse and Neglect* 11: 497–506.

Bok, S. (1982) *Secrets*, New York: Pantheon.

Briggs, S. (1987) 'The study of teachers' attitudes towards child sexual abuse', unpublished M.Sc. thesis, University of Glasgow.

Campis, L., Prentice-Dunn, S. and Lyman, R. (1989) 'Coping appraisal and parents' intentions to inform their children about sexual abuse: a protection motivation theory analysis', *Journal of Social and Clinical Psychology* 8, 3: 304–16.

Conte, J. R., Rosen, C. and Saperstein, L. (1986) 'An analysis of programmes to prevent the sexual victimisation of young children', *Journal of Primary Prevention* 6: 141–55.

deYoung, M. (1988) 'The good touch/bad touch dilemma', *Child Welfare* 67: 60–8.

Educational Media International, 235 Imperial Drive, Rayners Lane, Middlesex HA2 7HE.

Finkelhor, D. (1984) *Child Sexual Abuse: New Theory and Research*, London: Collier Macmillan.

Finkelhor, D. and Strapko, N. (1992) 'Sexual abuse prevention education: a review of evaluation studies', in D. Willis, E. Holden and M. Rosenberg (eds) *Prevention of Child Maltreatment: Developmental and Ecological Perspectives*, New York: Wiley.

Fotheringham, J. (1988) 'Sexual abuse: the teacher's perspective', in *Professional Development Initiatives 1987–88*, SED Regional Psychological Services.

Fryer, G., Kraizer, S. and Miyoshi, T. (1987) 'Measuring actual reduction of risk to child abuse: a new approach', *Child Abuse and Neglect* 11: 173–9.

Hazzard, A., Webb, C., Kleemeier, C., Angert, L. and Pohl, J. (1991) 'Child sexual abuse prevention: evaluation and one-year follow up', *Child Abuse and Neglect* 15: 123–38.

Kidscape, 82 Brook Street, London W1Y 1YG.

Kraizer, S.K. (1986) 'Rethinking prevention', *Child Abuse and Neglect* 10: 259–61.

Macleod, L. (1994) 'Parents as educators in the prevention of child sexual abuse', unpublished M.Phil. thesis, University of Strathclyde.

Mayes, G., Gillies, J. and Warden, D. (1990) 'An evaluation of the Kidscape Safety Training Programme', Research Report to the Scottish Office Education Department, Edinburgh: SOED publication.

Mayes, G., Currie, E., Macleod, L., Gillies, J. and Warden, D. (1992) *Child Sexual Abuse: A Review of Literature and Educational Materials*, Edinburgh: Scottish Academic Press.

Mayes, G., Gillies, J. and Warden, D. (1993) 'Stranger-danger: the development of children's understanding and constructs', Research Report to the Economic and Social Research Council.

Melton, G. (1992) 'The improbability of prevention of sexual abuse', in D. Willis, E. Holden and M. Rosenberg (eds) *Prevention of Child Maltreatment: Developmental and Ecological Perspectives*, New York: Wiley.

Pipe, M. and Goodman, G. (1991) 'Elements of secrecy: implications for children's testimony', *Behavioural Sciences and the Law* 9: 33–41.

Plummer, C. (1984) 'Preventing sexual abuse: what in-school programmes teach children', unpublished MSS, available from author at PO Box 421, Kalamazoo, MI 49005-0421, USA.

Reppucci, N. D. and Haugaard, J. J. (1989) 'Prevention of child sexual abuse: myth or reality', *American Psychologist* 44: 1266–75.

Rogers, R. W. (1983) 'Cognitive and physiological processes in fear appeals and attitude change: a revised theory of protection motivation', in J. T. Cacioppo and R. E. Petty (eds) *Social Psychophysiology: A Sourcebook*, New York: Guilford Press.

Rotter, J. B. (1982) *The Development and Application of Social Learning Theory*, New York: Praeger.

Scottish Office Home and Health Department, St Andrews House, Edinburgh EH1 3DE.

Tutty, L. M. (1992) 'The ability of elementary school children to learn child sexual abuse prevention concepts', *Child Abuse and Neglect* 16: 369–84.

Warden, D., Gillies, J. and Mayes, G. (in preparation) 'Children's conceptions of secrets'. Final report to ESRC.

Whiten, A. (1991) *Natural Theories of Mind*, Blackwell: Oxford.

Wurtele, S. K. (1987) 'School-based sexual abuse prevention programs', *Child Abuse and Neglect* 11: 483–95.

Wurtele, S. K. and Miller-Perrin, C. (1987) 'An evaluation of side-effects associated with participation in a child sexual abuse prevention programme', *Journal of School Health*, 57: 228–31.

Wurtele, S. K., Gillispie, E., Currier, L. and Franklin, C. (1992) 'A comparison of teachers versus parents as intructors of a personal safety program for pre-schoolers', *Child Abuse and Neglect* 16: 127–37.

Chapter 10

Bullying as a social problem in schools

James Boyle

In 1983 the Norwegian Ministry of Education established a nationwide anti-bullying campaign following two suicides adjudged to have been the direct result of bullying. Representatives from thirteen European countries attended a seminar on bullying held in Norway in 1987 under the aegis of the Council of Europe and interest grew as a result of recognition of the severity of the problems and evidence that something could be done about them (Munthe and Roland, 1989). This has led to an expansion of research and a move away from the traditional stance of regarding bullying as an inevitable part of 'growing up' which helps children learn to 'look after themselves', towards attempts to increase our understanding of bullying behaviour and how to deal with it (Tattum, 1993).

This chapter will examine the problems of defining and measuring the prevalence of bullying in schools and will consider the contribution of research to our understanding of the nature of the problem, its causes and effects. Research findings relating to the prevention and management of bullying in schools will be considered in Chapter 11.

DEFINING THE PROBLEM

The earliest empirical studies of the problems of bullying in schools were carried out in Sweden by Heinemann (1973 – see Roland, 1993) and Olweus (1978).

Heinemann (1973) originally used the term 'mobbing' to define the problem as he saw it, namely violent attacks on an individual, who is in some way deviant, by a *group* of perpetrators. However, this approach proved too restrictive in the light of subsequent studies which identified the prevalence of incidents of bullying involving individual perpetrators (Olweus, 1978). Olweus (1991: 413) offers the general definition:

A person is being bullied when he or she is exposed, repeatedly and over time, to negative actions on the part of one or more persons.

However, the phrase *negative actions* fails to make explicit the link between bullying and aggression highlighted in other definitions, such as that of Roland (1989: 21):

> Bullying is long-standing violence, physical or psychological, conducted by an individual or a group and directed against an individual who is not able to defend himself in the actual situation.

And of Besag (1989: 4):

> Bullying is a behaviour which can be defined as the repeated attack – physical, psychological, social or verbal – by those in a position of power, which is formally or situationally defined, on those who are powerless to resist, with the intention of causing distress for their own gain or gratification.

The above definitions incorporate four elements common to many others (see Johnstone *et al.*, 1992; Department for Education, 1994):

- that bullying behaviour involves wilful acts deliberately intended to hurt the victim and cause stress (Tattum, 1989);
- the view that bullying is not a 'one-off' incident, but rather is 'long-standing': repeated often and sustained over a period of time;
- that bullying need not involve *physical aggression* solely (e.g. hitting, kicking, tripping, theft, extortion etc.): it may be *verbal* (e.g. teasing, taunting, sexist or racist name-calling, spreading malicious stories etc.) or *psychological* (e.g. intimidation, social exclusion or gestures which imply later physical violence);
- that all types of bullying are forms of aggression involving an imbalance of power, with perpetrators illegitimately abusing their power over victims who are not able to defend themselves.

The imbalance of power which the perpetrator holds over the helpless victim and the level of distress which results is often used to differentiate bullying from other acts of aggression such as fighting (Roland, 1989). However, distinguishing between, say, teasing (which is commonly regarded as acceptable behaviour) and bullying can be more difficult (Pearce, 1991).

Olweus (1991: 413) provides a further useful distinction between *direct bullying*, consisting of 'open attacks upon the victim, either physical or verbal', and *indirect bullying*, consisting of exclusion or isolation from the group. Bullying thus can take many forms, many of them interrelated but all of them involving acts of aggression.

THE SCALE OF THE PROBLEM

A good deal of research in recent years has focused on measuring the prevalence, or frequency, of bullying problems in schools. However, the secretive nature of bullying and the lack of an accepted definition poses problems. Three approaches have been widely used: direct observation, reports from teachers or parents, and reports from children themselves (Smith and Sharp, 1994). Bullying tends to occur away from adult scrutiny and, as direct observation may thus be problematic, most surveys use indirect measures, such as interviews with teachers or pupils, self-report questionnaires (which may or may not be anonymous), and such other techniques as 'teacher nomination' and 'peer nomination'.

Teacher nomination

The earliest surveys of the prevalence of bullying in schools relied upon nominations from teachers of those pupils in their classes whom they believed to be involved in bully/victim problems. Table 10.1 provides details from three key studies which have used this approach.

The findings indicate considerable variation in prevalence rates. In Lowenstein's (1978a) survey 1.4 per cent of the pupils overall were identified as bullies compared to 5 per cent in Olweus' (1978) Swedish survey and 10 per cent in Stephenson and Smith's (1989) study of upper primary pupils in England, although the prevalence of bullies amongst boys of *secondary school age* in Lowenstein's study was 5 per cent, the same as in Olweus' sample of 13–15 year-olds. We shall consider factors which affect prevalence later in this section, but it is worth noting some of the advantages and disadvantages of the technique of teacher nomination. On the debit side, teachers are not always unanimous in their judgements as to what constitutes bullying behaviour and in any event seem to find it easier to identify victims rather than bullies (Lowenstein, 1978a; Siann *et al.*, 1993). School staff may not be aware of the full extent of bullying in their school because victims do not always tell their teachers about the problem. Stephenson and Smith (1989), for example, note that 22 per cent of victims reported that they never told their teachers about being bullied. However, although there is little information about the reliability (consistency) of the measure, studies indicate that the technique is valid, with significant correlations between teacher nominations and peer nominations ranging from 0.6–0.8 (Olweus, 1978; Perry *et al.*, 1988; Stephenson and Smith, 1989; Olweus, 1991).

Parent report

Reports from parents have also been used to estimate the prevalence of bullying. In their longitudinal study of child rearing in the UK, Newson and Newson (1984) found that the mothers of 25 per cent of their sample of 700 11-year-olds reported that their children were bullied in school, with 4 per cent being bullied seriously. The mothers also reported that a

Table 10.1 Prevalence of bully/victim problems: teacher nomination

Study	No. in sample	Age range	Prevalence
Olweus (1978): Sweden	1,000 boys	13–15 years	10% identified by their teachers as being involved in serious incidents of bullying, 5% as 'pronounced' bullies, and 5% as 'pronounced' victims. (With a less conservative criterion which included boys who showed only 'tendencies' towards being a bully or a victim, the overall level of involvement in bullying increased to 20%, with 10% of the boys as bullies and 10% as victims.) 3–7% of the boys were bully/victims
Lowenstein (1978a): England	5,774 children (2,858 males and 2,916 females) from 13 primary and 2 secondary schools	5–16 years	1.4% of children overall identified as bullies. But very stringent criteria to define bullying: the problems must have persisted for at least 6 months; and they had to be confirmed by 2 or more children, 2 or more teachers and by reports from victims or their parents
Stephenson and Smith (1989): England	1,078 pupils from 26 primary schools	10–11 years	Nominations from 49 teachers indicated that 23% of the children were involved in bullying, with 10% as bullies, 7% as victims, and 6% as bully/victims. Most of the bullying was long-term in nature, with 89% of the bullies and 72% of the victims reported to have been involved for at least a year

further 22 per cent of the children were bullied in the street. These levels of serious bullying are in line with those reported by Olweus (1978) and Lowenstein (1978a) above. However, as in the case of school staff, many parents and guardians are unaware that their children are being bullied because the children do not tell them, a problem which becomes more pronounced as children grow older. Studies carried out in the UK and Norway reveal that while around 55–65 per cent of victims of primary school age report telling their parents or guardians about being bullied, only 35–45 per cent of secondary school age disclose this to someone at home (Mellor, 1990; Whitney and Smith, 1993). Parent reports are thus likely to underestimate the prevalence of bullying, significantly so in the case of older pupils (Whitney and Smith, 1993), although the likelihood of telling a parent or guardian rises with the frequency of being bullied.

Pupil interviews

Elliott (1989) provided details of interviews carried out with 4,000 children aged between 5 and 16 years in the UK as part of the 'Kidscape' child protection initiative. Sixty-five per cent of the children overall reported being bullied, with 38 per cent reporting either being bullied twice or more or recounting a particularly terrifying experience of bullying. Of the children overall 3.8 per cent (3 per cent boys and 0.8 per cent girls) reported that long-term bullying was adversely affecting their everyday lives.

Interviews with children who are forthcoming about the problems can provide much useful information about the nature of bullying (see, for example, Junger's (1990) study of racial bullying in the Netherlands). But Ahmad and Smith (1990) note that the technique is less satisfactory in providing information about the prevalence of bullying problems because interviews are very time-consuming and do not reliably bring new cases to light since children can be defensive in an interview setting with an adult.

Peer nomination

The technique of peer nomination – asking pupils to identify those other children in their class who are the bullies or victims – is based on the premise that children themselves are the best able to judge who is involved in bully/victim problems. Children are not required to disclose their own involvement. In addition, the data obtained from a group of peers can be combined to increase the reliability of the scores and to minimise any effects of individual bias (Ahmad and Smith, 1990). Table 10.2 provides details from three key studies which have used this technique.

Table 10.2 Prevalence of bully/victim problems: peer nomination

Study	No. in sample	Age range	Prevalence
Bjorkqvist et al. (1982): Finland	401 pupils from three secondary schools	14–16 years	10.5% of the children were rated as being involved in bullying, 6.3% as bullies and 4.2% as victims
Perry et al. (1988): USA	165 pupils (83 boys and 82 girls) from one primary school	9–12 years	10% of the children were victims of serious physical bullying or verbal abuse by peers
Boulton and Smith (1994): England	158 children (83 boys and 75 girls) from three urban primary schools	8–9 years	35% of the children reported being involved in bullying, 13% as bullies, 17% as victims and 4.4% as both bullies and victims

The findings again reveal considerable variation in prevalence rates, with twice as many pupils in Florida being identified as being victims as in Finland, and higher levels still reported by Boulton and Smith (1994) in England. As we have seen, peer nominations are a valid means of establishing the identities of bullies or victims in a class and correlate significantly with teacher nominations. However, Ahmad and Smith (1990) note that peer nominations show higher levels of agreement with pupil self-report questionnaire data than do teacher nominations and hence may be a more satisfactory means of establishing prevalence, although perhaps less efficient in terms of time than self-report questionnaires.

Self-report questionnaires

Self-report questionnaires are currently by far the most commonly used technique for determining the extent of bully/victim problems in schools. Most studies have used variants of Olweus' *Bully/Victim Questionnaire* (see Olweus, 1991) and require pupils to respond anonymously to around 20 items relating to the form and prevalence of bullying, where it occurs, whether it has been reported (and to whom), and their own feelings about it. They are not required to identify other pupils as bullies or victims but instead are asked to indicate whether they themselves have ever bullied others or been the victim of bullying. The questionnaires are usually – though not always – administered by someone other than the usual class teacher and pupils are generally provided with definitions of bullying, such as the following based upon Olweus', and used in the largest survey carried out in England:

> We say a child or young person is being bullied, or picked on when another child or young person, or a group of children or young people, say nasty and unpleasant things to him or her. It is also bullying when a child or young person is hit, kicked, threatened, locked inside a room, sent nasty notes, when no one ever talks to them and things like that. These things can happen frequently and it is difficult for the child or the young person being bullied to defend himself or herself. It is also bullying when a child or young person is teased repeatedly in a nasty way. But it is not bullying when two children or young people of about the same strength have the odd fight or quarrel.
>
> (Whitney and Smith, 1993: 7)

Table 10.3 summarises the findings from ten studies which have used self-report questionnaires. This technique generally yields higher prevalence rates than the others, supporting the view that the results may be more valid, given the problems of denial by bullies and victims alike (Ahmad and Smith, 1990). However, although self-report data correlate

Table 10.3 Prevalence of bully/victim problems: self-report questionnaires

Study	No. in sample	Age range	Prevalence
Fonseca et al. (1989): Spain	1,200 pupils from 10 primary schools	8–12 years	17.3% reported bullying others during the current school term and 17.2% to being bullied. 12.7% experienced physical aggression and 19.3% being laughed at or teased. (No data are provided regarding the persistence of these problems)
O'Moore and Hillery (1989): Ireland	783 children (285 boys and 498 girls) from 4 primary schools	7–13 years	Around 55% of the pupils reported being victims occasionally and 43% were involved as bullies occasionally. 10.5% of the pupils were involved in bullying 'once a week' or more (8% as victims and 2.5% as bullies). Questionnaires were anonymous but administered by class teachers
Mellor (1990): Scotland	942 pupils from 10 secondary schools	12–16 years	10% involved in bullying 'sometimes or more often' (6% as victims and 4% as bullies, with 3% both bully and victim). 5% involved 'once a week or more often' (3% as victims and 2% as perpetrators). 50% of the pupils reported being involved in bullying at some time as victims, while 44% admitted to being perpetrators. 32% indicated that they had never been involved in bullying but 25% reported being involved in bullying 'sometimes or more often'
Olweus (1991): Norway	83,330 pupils from 404 schools	8–16 years	15% overall involved in bullying 'now and then or more often' (9% as victims, 7% as bullies and 1.6% as bully/victims). 5% involved in problems of bullying 'once per week or more' (3% as victims and 2% as bullies)
Rigby and Slee (1991): Australia	685 children from 3 primary and 1 secondary schools	6–16 years	6.1% of boys and 4.8% of girls identified themselves by means of self-reports as being 'picked on' by other pupils 'very often'

Study	Sample	Age	Findings
Boulton and Underwood (1992): England	296 pupils (154 boys and 142 girls) from 3 middle schools	8–9 11–12 years	21% reported being bullied, and 17% reported bullying others 'sometimes or more often'. 10% of the pupils reported being involved in bullying 'several times a week' (6.1% as victims and 3.8% as bullies)
Leslie (1993): Scotland	1,382 pupils (740 boys and 642 girls) from 7 primary schools	8–12 years	24.8% of the pupils reported being victims 'sometimes' while 3.1% of the children reported bullying others 'sometimes'. 8% of the children reported involvement in bullying on a weekly basis, 7% as victims and 0.8% as bullies, with 1.2% of the children reported being bullied on a daily basis
Mooij (1993): the Netherlands	1,065 pupils from 30 primary schools and 1,053 pupils from 36 secondary schools	9–10 11–12 13–14 15–16 years	43% of the primary pupils reported being involved in bullying 'now and then or more often', 23% as victims and 20% as bullies, compared to 22% of the secondary pupils (6% as victims and 16% as perpetrators). 14% of the primary pupils reported involvement in bullying 'once per week' (8% as victims and 6% as bullies) compared to 7% of secondary pupils (2% as victims and 5% as bullies). 7% of the primary school pupils reported being bullied several times per week (4% as victims and 3% as bullies) compared with 5% of secondary pupils (2% as victims and 3% as bullies)
Whitney and Smith (1993): England	6,758 pupils (3,423 boys and 3,335 girls) from 17 junior/middle and 7 secondary schools	8–16 years	39% of primary pupils reported involvement 'sometimes' in bullying (28% as victims and 12% as bullies). 14% of primary pupils reported being involved 'once a week or more' (10% as victims and 4% as bullies). 16% of secondary pupils reported being involved 'sometimes', in bullying (10% as victims and 6% as bullies). 5% reported involvement 'once per week or more' (4% as victims and 1% as bullies)
McLean (1994): Scotland	2,500 upper primary pupils (from 35 schools) and 7,500 secondary pupils (from 25 schools)	10–14 years	Pupils were invited to provide their own definitions of bullying. Around 20% reported personal involvement with bullying, with 53% reporting bullying as a serious problem in their schools. 4% of pupils reported being bullied every day, with 6% reporting being bullied for years

highly with the other methods discussed so far, there is still uncertainty about the reliability of the technique (Farrington, 1993).

DISCUSSION

The results from these surveys reveal considerable variation in the rates of reported bullying, with large differences across studies overall but also marked differences in the prevalence of bullying *between schools* in the same studies. The findings need interpretation in the light of factors which affect measures of prevalence:

- *How bullying is defined* Due to the absence of an agreed definition, bullying is defined in different ways across surveys. This is most evident in the case of criteria based upon the frequency of occurrences of bully/victim problems over time. Self-report questionnaires typically ask children to report whether bullying has occurred over the course of the present term: 'not at all', 'once or twice', 'sometimes' (or 'now and then'), 'once a week' or 'several times a week'. Clearly, the more conservative the criterion in terms of frequency of bullying, the lower the prevalence rates. This can be seen in the case of the studies reported in Table 10.3, where high proportions of pupils – usually around 15–20 per cent, although twice these rates in the case of some English studies (Whitney and Smith, 1993) – report involvement in bullying 'sometimes' during the course of a term, but only some 5–10 per cent report involvement on a more regular basis of 'once per week or more often'. Farrington argues that aggressive behaviour which occurs only once or twice should not, strictly speaking, be regarded as bullying, although it is interesting to note that studies which have considered *children's* perceptions of bullying (e.g. La Fontaine, 1991; McLean, 1994) have shown that many children regard 'one-off' or short-term incidents of aggression as bullying.

  The use of the 'school term' as the base time period for establishing prevalence rates also poses problems, as it can vary from 1–3 months depending upon when the study was carried out. It is clear that greater agreement regarding the frequency and persistence of 'serious' bullying and the time period used as the basis for measurement are required to permit meaningful comparisons between studies.
- *The method used to collect the data* As we have seen, a number of techniques have been used by researchers to estimate the prevalence of the problems of bullying, and we have considered evidence relating to their validity. But as Farrington (1993) notes, we still do not know enough about the reliability and validity of these measures. One of the major problems affecting reliability (i.e. the consistency of the measures) is that of response bias: the fact that pupils' responses can be

altered by the way in which the questions are framed. Ahmad and Smith (1990) provide evidence for this with their finding that more perpetrators were prepared to admit to bullying when an anonymous questionnaire was used than 'on the record' in an interview. Siann *et al.* (1994) also note the importance of contextual variables such as the effects of the questions preceding those directly concerned with bullying upon pupils' responses.

A number of studies consider reliability in terms of the 'percentage of agreement between different measures' (e.g. see Olweus, 1978; Ahmad and Smith, 1990). However, this is not as satisfactory a measure of reliability as comparing test and re-test scores across a short time interval (Rust and Golombok, 1989). Without this kind of information about reliability it is difficult to evaluate whether a 5 per cent prevalence rate of bullying in one study is significantly lower than, say, a 9 per cent rate in a second, or even more fundamentally, whether bullying is on the increase (Olweus, 1991). We shall also see in the next chapter that it poses marked problems for attempts to determine the success of intervention programmes.

- *The age and gender of the pupils* Findings from the large-scale studies summarised in Table 10.3 indicate that while the percentage of perpetrators remains fairly constant as pupils become older, the percentage of those bullied decreases markedly with the pupils' age (Olweus, 1991; Whitney and Smith, 1993). This results in problems in generalising survey findings across considerably different age-ranges and also poses problems for comparison of results from surveys carried out at different times of the year (Smith, 1994). There are also problems in generalising across gender. For example, Olweus (1991) notes that boys are more likely to be involved in bully/victim problems: three times as many boys as girls are bullies overall and twice as many boys as girls are victims. He also reports that the prevalence of female bullies declines steadily with age but prevalence of male bullies remains roughly the same between 8–16 years. In addition, boys tend to be involved more in direct, physical bullying than girls, who engage more in verbal and indirect, psychological bullying (Whitney and Smith, 1993). However, Roland (1989) suggests that such gender differences may be the result of response bias, with girls being less willing than boys to admit to being involved in violent interactions.
- *The opportunities available within the school for bullying to take place* Increasing 'teacher density' (or supervision) at breaks reduces the opportunities for bullying and is associated with lower prevalence rates (Olweus, 1993). The levels of supervision by staff in a school can markedly affect the levels of bullying.
- *The sensitivity of staff, pupils and parents to the problems of bullying* Increasing the awareness of staff, pupils and parents to the problems

of bullying, particularly as part of a 'whole-school policy' can also help to reduce the prevalence in school.

(Olweus, 1991; Smith and Sharp, 1994)

The surveys reviewed here indicate that bullying is a significant problem in schools. Around 20 per cent of pupils overall may have some personal involvement in bullying, although the rate in some urban primary schools may be twice as high as this. But the problems are of a persistent and serious nature for around 5–10 per cent. Generally, the rates of bully/victim problems in England, Ireland and the Netherlands appear to be higher than in Norway and Scotland, perhaps because of the extent to which the studies have been carried out in inner-city areas.

Although some 60–70 per cent of pupils appear to be uninvolved in bullying, studies indicate high levels of awareness of the problems of bullying amongst pupils as a whole. As Arora and Thompson (1987) put it, bullying is a 'known secret' amongst peers and in the next chapter we shall consider how the problems of bullying can be addressed by utilising the resources of those who are uninvolved to help develop more positive social relations in schools. Siann *et al.* (1994) note that establishing the prevalence of bullying hinges on a subjective process of 'social construction' involving labelling complex social interactions and attributing intentionality. It is unlikely, therefore, that the use of a single, coarse-grained technique such as a self-report questionnaire will capture all of the complexities involved. Farrington (*op. cit.*) points out that greater use should be made of direct observation of playground behaviour, for example. But it is also clear that more detailed information about how different techniques of measuring bullying relate is required, particularly as different approaches may provide similar estimates of overall prevalence rate but base these upon the identification of different children.

THE NATURE OF THE PROBLEM

Bullying tends to occur most commonly in settings where the level of adult supervision is low, typically in the playground in primary and secondary schools (Olweus, 1991; Whitney and Smith, 1993). However, it also occurs frequently in classrooms and corridors in secondary schools (Mellor, 1990; Whitney and Smith, 1993). Bullying also takes place more frequently in school than on the journey to and from home though those bullied on their way to school tended also to be bullied in school (Olweus, 1991).

Whitney and Smith note that the most common forms of bullying are name-calling (which accounted for 50 per cent of incidents in primaries and 62 per cent in secondaries in Whitney and Smith's sample), physical violence (26 per cent), being threatened (25 per cent), or having rumours spread (24 per cent). Having personal belongings taken (10 per cent), racial harassment (9 per cent) and social exclusion or 'being sent to Coventry' (7 per cent) were less commonly reported. The prevalence of bullying does not appear to be associated with the ethnic mix in schools and there is no indication that children from ethnic backgrounds are more likely to be bullied or to be bullies (Junger, 1990; Olweus, 1991; Moran *et al.*, 1993; Whitney and Smith, 1993), although Siann *et al.* (1994) note some ethnic differences in the way that children label problems as bullying.

Bullying behaviour does not appear to be linked to the size of school (Olweus, 1991; Whitney and Smith, 1993) although *size of class* in secondary schools was associated with more serious problems of bullying in Whitney and Smith's study. However, there is a significant association between social disadvantage and bullying (Stephenson and Smith, 1989).

As we have seen, bully/victim problems become less prevalent as children become older and there are significant gender differences: the percentage of victims declines sharply with age and the percentage of female bullies declines steadily with age, but the percentage of male bullies remains broadly the same between 8 and 16 years.

In general, boys bully more than girls although boys and girls are equally victimised. Boys are usually bullied by boys, mainly by one child at a time (in 55 per cent of cases), though bullying by several boys (29 per cent) and by mixed groups (12 per cent) are not uncommon (Whitney and Smith, 1993). Bullying by groups of pupils may bring to bear additional mechanisms which serve to diffuse the individual responsibility, weaken control over aggression and reduce empathy with the victim (Olweus, 1978). Perpetrators often turn their attentions onto more than one victim and Stephenson and Smith (1989) note that 67 per cent of the bullies in their study victimised more than one pupil at a given time, with 78 per cent of the victims being bullied by different children.

However, it is rare for a boy to be bullied by a girl acting on her own. Girls almost invariably bully only other girls (Olweus, 1991). On the other hand, girls tend to be bullied by both boys and girls. The majority of bullies are in the same class or year as their victims, although around 30 per cent of bullies (chiefly in primary schools) are older (Whitney and Smith, 1993). McLean (1994) notes that boys in particular are more likely to be bullied by older pupils.

Boys tend to bully and be bullied both directly and indirectly, whereas girls are more likely to bully and be bullied indirectly, using social exclusion and harmful gossip (Olweus, 1991). The rates of indirect bullying are broadly the same for boys and girls (Stephenson and Smith, 1989) and boys are thus subject to additional physical aggression which may serve as a means for the bully to achieve power and status within the peer group. Whitney and Smith (1993) note that 54 per cent of primary pupils and 34 per cent of secondary pupils indicate that they tried to help pupils whom they saw being bullied. However, 16 per cent of primary and 25 per cent of secondary pupils reported that they would join in with the bullying.

Bully/victim problems are more prevalent in schools and classes for pupils with special educational needs (O'Moore and Hillery, 1989; Stephenson and Smith, 1989). Pupils with special needs who are integrated into mainstream schools are also particularly vulnerable with regard to bullying, largely because they are less popular and more likely to be socially rejected (Whitney *et al.*, 1992; Nabuzoka and Smith, 1993). However, personal characteristics such as physically handicapping conditions or obesity are not strongly associated with the incidence of bullying, although victims tend to be physically weaker than their peers (Lowenstein, 1978b; Olweus 1978; 1991).

The problems of bullying tend to persist over time. Olweus (1978) found considerable stability of bullies and victims of secondary school age using peer ratings after a 3-year follow-up. Similar findings are reported by Boulton and Smith (1994). However, as Stephenson and Smith (1989) note, the problems need not be continuous: there were occasions when three-quarters of the bullies and victims in their study were not involved in bully/victim problems.

'BULLIES AND VICTIMS'

Studies of bullies and victims have tended to focus upon personality characteristics, and less importance has been given to the group dynamics underpinning the problems (Roland, 1993). Studies such as that of Olweus (1978) and Stephenson and Smith (1989) indicate that bullies tend to be highly aggressive, impulsive, physically strong (in the case of males), and to have marked needs for power and dominance over others. They tend to have positive attitudes towards violence and aggression and have little regard for their victims. Bullies are often out-going and confident, with good self-esteem, and in the main do not present as insecure or anxious. In general they do not appear to feel guilt about their bullying. However, there are a small number of 'anxious' bullies (perhaps around 18 per cent of all bullies, according to Stephenson and Smith) who lack confidence and join in bullying instigated by others (see also Whitney and Smith, 1993). Bullies tend to be of average or just below average popularity, although they become less popular with age. Male bullies are often of slightly below-average intelligence and low school attainments and tend to have negative attitudes towards school work and teachers. However, female bullies are often more intelligent and may experience above-average levels of academic success in school (Roland, 1989).

In contrast, victims tend to be anxious, insecure, passive, with low self-esteem (Bjorkqvist *et al.*, 1982; Boulton and Smith, 1994), and if boys,

tend to be physically weaker than their peers (Olweus, 1978). They commonly see themselves as having little worth and are often lonely and
socially isolated in school. They show high levels of anxiety in social
interactions and have difficulties in assertion in the playground. They
tend to be unpopular and are rejected by their peers (Perry *et al.*, 1988).
The extent to which physical characteristics increase the likelihood of
being a victim is unclear (Olweus, 1978; Besag, 1989) although a lack of
physical attractiveness may add to the risk (Lowenstein, 1978b; Stephenson
and Smith, 1989).

Bjorkquist *et al.* (1982) suggest that cognitive changes on the part of
bullies and victims alike may be used to justify and hence sustain persistent bullying. For example, bullies may interpret the behaviour of their
victims as provocative or aggressive (Boulton and Underwood, 1992),
and victims as a result of their low self-esteem, may start to believe that
they 'deserve' it (Roland, 1989).

There have been a number of attempts to identify sub-groups of victims.
A convincing case can be made for a group of 'provocative' victims
(perhaps 17 per cent of all victims, according to Stephenson and Smith,
1989), who are characterised by high levels of aggression and anxiety
(Olweus, 1978). They are commonly restless, active children, who have
problems with concentration and behave in irritating ways which can
lead to negative reactions from a whole class. More controversial are the
'bully-victims' (Stephenson and Smith, 1989) who can be both bullies and
victims, depending upon circumstances, although they do not usu- ally
bully those children who bully them. Farrington (1993) notes that as
many as 38 per cent of bullies may also be victims, and 46 per cent of
victims may also be bullies, highlighting the need for more research into
the overlap.

Longitudinal research studies reveal that persistent male bullies are
four times as likely to have had three or more court convictions at age 24
(Olweus, 1991). And in a similar vein, former victims report continuing
problems of depression and low self-esteem at age 23 which may adversely affect adult relationships (Olweus, 1993). Farrington (1993) reports
on the findings of a 24-year longitudinal study and notes that boys who
bully at age 14 also tend to bully at age 32, indicating considerable
'intragenerational continuity' amongst those who bully. However, he also
presents evidence for 'intergenerational continuity', of the specific transmission of bullying across a generation: the boys who bullied at 14 tended
themselves at age 32 to have children who bullied. However, most longitudinal, prospective studies have followed up male bullies and there is a
need for more research into the outcomes for females, particularly female
bullies.

There has been considerable interest in identifying factors which cause
such persistent problems of bullying. As we have seen, temperament and

personality variables such as marked (and poorly controlled) aggressive tendencies and impulsivity are associated with bullying behaviour, and passivity, low self-esteem and lack of assertion are associated with victimisation. Socio-economic factors in themselves do not appear to be specifically related to bullying but the quality of parental relationships and use of physical punishment in the home are judged to be significant risk factors (Olweus, 1978). Olweus (1984) reports that maternal indifference, a permissive approach to discipline, and parental use of physical punishment were associated with high levels of displays of aggressive behaviour across many different situations in Swedish boys aged 13–16 years. The role of fathers was found to be less crucial, perhaps reflecting a relative lack of involvement. In contrast, over-protective parenting may increase the risk factor of a child becoming a victim, by reducing the opportunities for the child to develop age-appropriate skills of independence and self-assertion (Olweus, 1993). Bowers, Smith and Binney (1992) confirm the influences of family dynamics (in the form of perceptions of power and cohesion) upon bullies, victims, and bully/victims, but more research exploring the group dynamics of bully–victim interaction in school settings is required.

CONCLUDING COMMENTS

This chapter has considered the problems of defining and measuring bullying, together with research findings regarding the nature of bullying and the characteristics of bullies and their victims. Around 10 per cent of pupils on average may be regarded as being involved in long-standing, serious problems either as victim or bully. However, we have identified a need for higher levels of agreement regarding the definition of bullying, particularly with regard to the time base for definitions, together with a greater emphasis upon the reliability of measures of the prevalence of bullying. Improvements of this kind would clarify issues such as the suggestion that bullying has become more common. Farrington (1993) also emphasises the need for longitudinal study of bullies and victims, particularly of the long-term outcomes of bullying for females, which could inform the direction of preventive intervention strategies.

An adequate understanding of bullying thus requires more than just consideration of the personality characteristics of bullies and victims. The degree of overlap between bullies and victims reported in recent studies alone indicates the limitations of this traditional approach and highlights the importance of the *context* in which bullying occurs and of the nature of the *interactions* between bullies, victims and bystanders. As Stainton Rogers (1991: 6) puts it, 'Bullies create victims and victims create bullies'. Bullying thus cannot be regarded as a set of inflexible categories of 'bullies' and 'victims', and cannot be 'cured' just by treating the victim

(Mellor, 1991). There is a pressing need, therefore, to build upon empirical studies of the relationship between aggressive behaviour and peer status in children's social interactions (e.g. Coie *et al.*, 1991).

'Bullying' in schools can be regarded therefore as the outcome of complex processes of social interaction which are generally controlled by the bully, while the majority of pupils remain bystanders, uninvolved but aware of the difficulties (Smith and Sharp, 1994). Traditionally, some schools tended to ignore bullying, but the situation has changed dramatically in the light of public concern about the effects upon bullies and victims alike and concern by teachers about the damaging effects of bullying upon school ethos. This has led to increased interest in identifying effective ways of managing and preventing the problems of bullying which we shall consider in the next chapter.

REFERENCES

Ahmad, Y. S. and Smith, P. K. (1990) 'Behavioural measures review no. 1: bullying in schools', *Newsletter of the Association for Child Psychology and Psychiatry* 12: 26–7.

Arora, C. M. J. and Thompson, D. A. (1987) 'Defining bullying for a secondary school', *Education and Child Psychology* 4: 110–20.

Besag, V. (1989) *Bullies and Victims in Schools: A Guide to Understanding and Management*, Buckingham: Open University Press.

Bjorkqvist, K., Ekman, K. and Lagerspetz, K. (1982) 'Bullies and victims: their ego picture, ideal ego picture and normative ego picture', *Scandinavian Journal of Psychology* 23: 307–13.

Boulton, M. J. and Underwood, K. (1992) 'Bully victim problems among middle-school children', *British Journal of Educational Psychology* 62, 1: 73–87.

Boulton, M. J. and Smith, P. K. (1994) 'Bully/victim problems in middle-school children: stability, self-perceived competence, peer perceptions and peer acceptance', *British Journal of Developmental Psychology* 12: 315–29.

Bowers, L., Smith, P. K. and Binney, V. (1992) 'Cohesion and power in the families of children involved in bully/victim problems in schools', *Journal of Family Therapy* 14: 371–87.

Byrne, B. (1994) *Coping with Bullying in Schools*, London: Cassell.

Coie, J. D., Dodge, K. A., Terry, R. and Wright, V. (1991) 'The role of aggression in peer relationships: an analysis of aggression episodes in boys play groups', *Child Development* 62: 812–26.

DES (1989) *Discipline in Schools (The Elton Report)*, London: HMSO

Department for Education (1994) *Bullying: Don't Suffer in Silence. An Anti-bullying Pack for Schools*, London: HMSO.

Elliott, M. (1989) 'Bullying – harmless fun or murder', in E. Munthe and E. Roland (eds) *Bullying: An International Perspective*, London: David Fulton.

Farrington, D. P. (1993) 'Understanding and preventing bullying', in M. Tonry (ed.) *Crime and Justice: A Review of Research Vol. 17*, Chicago: The University of Chicago Press.

Fonseca, M. M. V., Garcia, I. F. and Perez, G. Q. (1989) 'Violence, bullying and counselling in the Iberian Peninsula', in E. Munthe and E. Roland (eds) *Bullying: An International Perspective*, London: David Fulton.

Heinemann, P. P. (1973) *Mobbing: gruppevold blant barn og voksne (Bullying: Group-violence among Children and Adults)*, Oslo: Gyldendal.

Johnstone, M., Munn, P. and Edwards, L. (1992) *Action against Bullying: A Support Pack for Schools*, Edinburgh: Scottish Council for Research in Education.

Junger, M. (1990) 'Intergroup bullying and racial harassment in the Netherlands', *Sociology and Social Research* 74: 65–72.

La Fontaine, J. (1991) *Bullying: The Child's View*, London: Calouste Gulbenkian Foundation.

Leslie, B. (1993) 'Bullying in Scottish primary schools: a survey of bullying in seven Scottish primary schools', unpublished M.Sc. dissertation, University of Strathclyde.

Lowenstein, L. F. (1978a) 'Who is the bully?', *Bulletin of the British Psychological Society* 31: 147–9.

—— (1978b) 'The bullied and non-bullied child', *Bulletin of the British Psychological Society* 31: 316–18.

McLean, A. V. (1994) *Bullying Survey in Strathclyde Region*, Glasgow North East Psychological Service, Strathclyde Regional Council.

Mellor, A. (1990) *Bullying in Scottish Secondary Schools*, SCRE Spotlights Number 23, Edinburgh: SCRE.

—— (1991) 'Helping victims', in M. Elliott (ed.) *Bullying: A Practical Guide to Coping for Schools*, Harlow, Essex: Longman.

Mooij, T. (1993) 'Working towards understanding and prevention in the Netherlands', in D. Tattum (ed.) *Understanding and Managing Bullying*, Oxford: Heinemann Educational.

Moran, S., Smith, P. K., Thompson, D. and Whitney, I. (1993) 'Ethnic differences in experiences of bullying – Asian and white children', *British Journal of Educational Psychology* 63, 3: 431–40.

Munthe, E. and Roland, E. (eds) (1989) *Bullying: An International Perspective*, London: David Fulton.

Nabuzoka, D. and Smith, P. K. (1993) 'Sociometric status and social behaviour of children with and without learning difficulties', *Journal of Child Psychology and Psychiatry*, 34, 8: 1435–48.

Newson, J. and Newson, E. (1984) 'Parents' perspectives on children's behaviour at school', in N. Frude and H. Gault (eds) *Disruptive Behaviour in Schools*, Chichester: John Wiley and Sons.

O'Moore, A. M. and Hillery, B. (1989) 'Bullying in Dublin schools', *Irish Journal of Psychology* 10, 3: 426–41.

—— (1991) 'What do teachers need to know?' in M. Elliott (ed.) *Bullying: A Practical Guide to Coping for Schools*, Harlow, Essex: Longman.

Olweus, D. (1978) *Aggression in the Schools: Bullies and Whipping Boys*, Washington: Hemisphere Publishing Corporation.

—— (1984) 'Aggressors and their victims: bullying at school', in N. Frude and H. Gault (eds) *Disruptive Behaviour in Schools*, Chichester: John Wiley and Sons.

—— (1991) 'Bully/victim problems among schoolchildren: basic facts and effects of a school based intervention program', in D. J. Pepler and K. H. Rubin (eds) *The Development and Treatment of Childhood Aggression*, Hillsdale, New Jersey: Lawrence Erlbaum Associates.

—— (1993) *Bullying at School: What We Know and What We Can Do*, Oxford: Blackwell.

—— (1994) 'Bullying at school: basic facts and effects of a school based intervention program', *Journal of Child Psychology and Psychiatry* 35, 7: 1171–90.

Pearce, J. (1991) 'What can be done about the bully?', in M. Elliott (ed.) *Bullying: A Practical Guide to Coping for Schools*, Harlow, Essex: Longman.

Perry, D. G., Kusel, S. J. and Perry, L. C. (1988) 'Victims of peer aggression', *Developmental Psychology* 24, 6: 807–14.

Rigby, K. and Slee, P. T. (1991) 'Bullying among Australian school-children: reported behaviour and attitudes towards victims', *Journal of Social Psychology* 131, 5: 615–27.

Roland, E. (1989) 'Bullying: the Scandinavian research tradition', in D. P. Tattum and D. A. Lane (eds) *Bullying in Schools*, Stoke-on-Trent: Trentham Books.

—— (1993) 'Bullying: a developing tradition of research and management', in D. Tattum (ed.) *Understanding and Managing Bullying*, Oxford: Heinemann Educational.

Rust, J. and Golombok, S. (1989) *Modern Psychometrics: The Science of Psychological Assessment*, London: Routledge.

Siann, G., Callaghan, M., Lockhart, R. and Rawson, L. (1993) 'Bullying: within school variables and the views of teachers', *Educational Studies* 19: 301–29.

Siann, G., Callaghan, M., Glissov, P., Lockhart, R. and Rawson, L. (1994) 'Who gets bullied? The effect of school, gender and ethnic group', *Educational Research* 36, 2: 123–34.

Smith, P. K. (1994) Personal communication.

Smith, P. K. and Sharp, S. (1994) 'The problem of school bullying', in P. K. Smith and S. Sharp (eds) *School Bullying: Insights and Perspectives*, London: Routledge.

Stainton Rogers, R. (1991) 'Now you see it, now I don't', in M. Elliott (ed.) *Bullying: A Practical Guide to Coping for Schools*, Harlow, Essex: Longman.

Stephenson, P. and Smith, D. (1989) 'Bullying in the junior school', in D. P. Tattum and D. A. Lane (eds) *Bullying in Schools*, Stoke-on-Trent: Trentham Books.

Tattum, D. (1989) 'Violence and aggression in schools', in D. P. Tattum and D. A. Lane (eds) *Bullying in Schools*, Stoke-on-Trent: Trentham Books.

—— (1993) *Understanding and Managing Bullying*, Oxford: Heinemann Educational.

Tattum, D. and Herbert, G. (1993) *Countering Bullying: Initiatives by Schools and Local Authorities*, Stoke-on-Trent: Trentham Books.

Whitney, I., Nabuzoka, D. and Smith, P. K. (1992) 'Bullying in schools: mainstream and special needs', *Support for Learning* 7, 1: 3–7.

Whitney, I. and Smith, P. K. (1993) 'A survey of the nature and extent of bullying in junior, middle and secondary schools', *Educational Research* 35, 1: 3–25.

Chapter 11

The management and prevention of bullying

James Boyle

The research reviewed in the previous chapter shows bullying to be a complex problem common to most schools, neglected until comparatively recently. Uncertainty as to how to deal with bullying behaviour was highlighted by Stephenson and Smith (1989) who found that 25 per cent of a sample of 49 teachers were reluctant to intervene for fear of exacerbating the problem. However, issues relating to the management and prevention of bullying have come to the fore in the UK in recent years. Key factors have been:

- the concern expressed by the media and public following suicides by pupils who had been victimised by bullies in schools (see Smith and Sharp, 1994a)
- the attention drawn to bullying by the 'Kidscape' child protection programme (Elliott, 1986; 1989)
- the dissemination of Scandinavian research into bullying (Olweus, 1984; Munthe, 1989; Munthe and Roland, 1989)
- the report of the Elton Committee on discipline in schools in England and Wales (Department of Education and Science, 1989) highlighting the adverse effects of bullying upon school atmosphere and the need to develop whole-school behaviour policies to tackle the problems of bullying and racial harassment
- the publication of the first books on the subject written by UK authors (e.g. Besag, 1989; Tattum and Lane, 1989) together with the first surveys of the prevalence of bullying in schools in the UK (Yates and Smith, 1989; Mellor, 1990)
- the working group set up by the Calouste Gulbenkian Foundation (UK Branch) in 1989 which provided funding for a wide range of initiatives such as:

  - an information booklet on bullying for schools (Tattum and Herbert, 1990)
  - a telephone helpline for children, the 'Bullying Line' (La Fontaine, 1991)

- anti-bullying materials for 'Kidscape' (see Elliott, 1991a)
- anti-bullying drama presentations (Gobey, 1991)
- funding for an investigation of the prevalence and nature of bullying behaviour in 24 schools in Sheffield and for a survey service for schools more generally (Ahmad *et al.*, 1991)
- a bibliography of resources and strategies for tackling bullying (Skinner, 1992)
- materials to help teachers develop whole-school anti-bullying policies (Besag, 1992; Tattum *et al.* 1993)
- a volume of case studies of anti-bullying initiatives (Tattum and Herbert, 1993)
- and a research project focusing on the environment of the playground (Higgins, 1994)

- the Sheffield Anti-Bullying Project which was set up with funding from the Department for Education to evaluate the effectiveness of the intervention strategies introduced in the schools in Sheffield which had been involved in the Gulbenkian-funded survey (see Whitney *et al.*, 1994a)
- the distribution of anti-bullying support packs to schools in the UK by government education departments (e.g. Johnstone *et al.*, 1992; Munn, 1993; Mellor, 1993; Department for Education, 1994)
- the publication of books written for teachers and parents which provide practical suggestions for dealing with bullying (e.g. Elliott, 1991b; Smith and Thompson, 1991; Olweus, 1993; Tattum, 1993a; Byrne, 1994; McLean, 1994; Sharp and Smith, 1994)

Hence a wealth of practical advice is currently available to schools and parents. But how should they proceed if they wish to address the problems of bullying? A first step is to make a functional distinction between the *management* and the *prevention* of bullying: that is, between measures designed to meet the need for immediate, direct action to respond effectively when an incident of bullying is uncovered or reported (i.e. crisis management), and longer-term intervention designed to reduce the likelihood of bullying occurring. Such approaches can be sub-divided in terms of intervention at the level of the *individual pupil*, at the level of the *class*, at the level of the *school* as a whole and indeed at the level of the *community* more generally (Stephenson and Smith, 1989).

In this chapter we consider first how the problems of bullying can be managed and controlled by schools at each of the above levels; then what steps schools might take to prevent bullying. Finally we review the evidence on the effectiveness of intervention, concluding with a discussion of the implications for practice and policy in schools.

THE MANAGEMENT OF BULLYING IN SCHOOLS

Intervention focused on known individuals involved in bullying falls into three categories: direct work with bullies; direct work with victims; and joint work with bullies and victims.

Direct work with bullies

As a first step, we need to clarify the nature of the bullying episodes. For example, if the perpetrator is an 'anxious' bully (i.e. unpopular, insecure, with poor educational attainment), then a management strategy which addresses the pupil's problems in self-confidence, self-esteem, social skills and school attainment may be more appropriate than one which focuses unduly upon sanctions. Similarly, if the bullying is carried out by a gang, then some of the group management strategies may be more effective than dealing with all of the bullies as individuals (Pikas, 1989). Particular problems such as racial and sexual harassment or the involvement of pupils with special educational needs should also be identified (Gillborn, 1993; Drouet, 1993; Whitney *et al.*, 1994b). And as a matter of course, the possibility of learning difficulties should be borne in mind for all pupils identified as bullies. In addition, the time, location and frequency of the bullying incidents should be noted as these may have implications for supervision.

Approaches typically used with bullies include sanctions; attempts to 'reason' and talk through the problems; developing empathy for the victim; rewarding desirable behaviour; and social skills training (Besag, 1989; Tattum, 1993b).

Sanctions: punishments and deterrents

Studies of school effectiveness reveal that poorer standards of pupil behaviour are in general associated with an undue emphasis upon punishment while better standards of behaviour are associated with generous use of praise and rewards (Rutter *et al.*, 1979; Mortimore *et al.*, 1988).

Foster and Thompson (1991) argue that the use of explicit physical punishments may legitimise aggression in the eyes of the bully and assert that effective sanctions should be non-violent and make use of the effects of peer pressure upon the bully.

An example of such an approach is the 'bully court', developed by Laslett (1982) to deal with the problems of bullying in a day school for primary school-aged children with emotional and behavioural difficulties. A small group of between two to five children are selected by their peers to hear complaints from victims in a court-like setting, with teacher representation, and administer punishments from a previously agreed list to bullies. Laslett reports that bully courts reduced the incidence of bullying in his school and that the bullies benefited from both the comments made by the other children and the punishment administered (for example being required to apologise and make some form of restitution, or losing privileges). Olweus (1991) is critical of the approach as it focuses on punishment rather than prevention and administers punishments long after the incidents of bullying, thus reducing their effectiveness. Smith *et al.* (1994c) also note that many teachers are resistant to the idea of bully courts in principle, as they are uncomfortable about having children 'judge' their classmates.

Elliott (1991c) reported a fall from 70 per cent to 6 per cent in pupils' reports of being bullied following the introduction of bully courts in eight schools. However, it is difficult to make a meaningful comparison between these data because of differences in the time period involved: the 70 per cent appears to refer to having been bullied 'at some time', whereas the 6 per cent refers to having been bullied in 'the last three months', a more conservative criterion.

In Brier and Ahmad's (1991) study anonymous self-report questionnaires were administered before and after bully courts were set up in a primary school. The results revealed falls of 7 per cent in the prevalence of being bullied and around 5 per cent in the prevalence of bullying which were in contrast to slight increases in the prevalence in uninvolved classes. However, as it would appear that the bully court only met on two occasions, the observed decrease in bullying may have been more to do with the groupwork activities and the other elements of the process of establishing the courts.

In conclusion, the case for bully courts is far from clear-cut. They are unlikely to be successful unless as a means of introducing intensive groupwork activities and in any event are very time-consuming to set up and are rarely used by schools. There are additional practical problems noted by Johnstone *et al.*, (1992), including the range of punishments available to the 'court', the appropriateness of the approach for dealing with gangs of bullies, and the acceptability of bully courts to the parents of bullies.

'Reasoning'

The survey carried out by Stephenson and Smith (1989) indicated that most of the teachers in their sample reported relying upon talk-based approaches to deal with bullies. Chazan (1989) and Frost (1991) also emphasise the importance of talking to bullies to communicate the inappropriate nature of their behaviour. There is little evidence that such methods are particularly effective with aggressive children (Topping, 1983) and the approaches do not utilise the effects of group dynamics and peer pressure. However, 'serious talks' between teachers and bullies expressing disapproval, stressing that bullying is unacceptable, and warning of sanctions for future misconduct are a key aspect of Olweus' (1993) multi-level intervention programme.

Developing empathy for victims

A number of writers such as Besag (1989), Priest (1989), Lowenstein (1991), Pearce (1991) and Tattum (1993b) recommend the use of counselling to help bullies increase their understanding of the victim's point of view and feelings. However, Coie et al. (1991) note that there is a lack of evidence from controlled studies to support the view that such 'perspective-taking' approaches are helpful with aggressive children. (Group approaches such as 'The Method of Common Concern' (Pikas, 1989) and the 'No Blame' method (Maines and Robinson, 1991) designed to encourage bullies to develop feelings of empathy for their victims by engaging bullies (and victims) in a group problem-solving process are discussed below.)

Behavioural approaches

Educational psychologists in Stephenson and Smith's (1989) study advocated the use of behavioural techniques to tackle the problems of bullying, particularly the reinforcement of more desirable, non-aggressive behaviour (e.g. by involving bullies as peer tutors). There has been little formal evaluation of the use of these approaches with individual bullies, but Coie et al. (1991) point out that such behavioural interventions can successfully reduce aggressive behaviour. Cognitive-behavioural approaches to impulse and anger control have also been evaluated, but with less clear-cut reduction in aggressive behaviour.

Social skills training

Social skills training is designed to help children and young people acquire more appropriate social behaviour and friendship skills by means of activities focused on the skills of interaction and social problem-solving skills, such as conflict resolution. Although research has been carried out on the use of social skills training with the victims of bullying (Arora, 1991), there has been comparatively little on the use of the approach with bullies per se. Coie et al. (1991) note that while there is evidence supporting the effectiveness of such training with aggressive children, there are problems with the transfer and generalisation of such skills to real-life situations, generally as a result of low motivation.

Newer theoretical approaches to conflict resolution and social problem-solving include solution-focused brief therapy (de Shazer, 1985), which encourages clients to focus upon their own perceptions of their needs and workable goals and to define their own solutions to their problem, with support from the therapist who suggests tasks to help them achieve these goals.However, little formal research has been carried out into the long-term effectiveness of this method with bullies.

Direct work with victims

As before, the nature of the problem, and the time, location and frequency of the bullying should be considered first. Stephenson and Smith (1989) note that it is important to distinguish 'provocative victims' (that is, those who are easily provoked and claim to be 'picked on') from the more typical 'passive' victims, as the provocative victims need the support of activities to help them accept that their behaviour is a causal factor in their experience of being bullied.

In general, direct work with victims in schools is of three kinds: discussions following the disclosure of bullying to ensure that teachers are fully aware of the nature and context of the problems; provision of peer support; and strategies to develop social skills (e.g. including assertiveness training to develop confidence and self-esteem) (Besag, 1989).

Discussions with teachers

Initial investigation of the bullying problem provides an opportunity not only for collecting factual information but also for the victim to be given reassurance that something is being done (Chazan, 1989). It is also important to emphasise the appropriateness of 'telling' teachers and parents about bullying to minimise any guilt the victim may feel as a result of disclosure (Mellor, 1991). Practical advice can also be given by teachers: for example, the importance of staying with a group; of not being alone in school toilets and changing rooms; of not bringing expensive toys or other valuables into school; and of trying not to show emotions in front of the bullies (Besag, 1989). Olweus (1993) also identifies 'serious talks' with victims as an important component of his intervention programme.

Peer support

Peer support can be provided in a number of ways, for example, by asking a classmate or older pupil to watch over the victim (Besag, 1989), or perhaps by means of 'peer counselling' (Sharp and Cowie, 1994), in which pupils are trained in basic counselling skills to provide a 'listening service' to those experiencing difficulties. However, the effectiveness of these approaches with the victims of bullying has yet to be established.

Social skills training

Arora (1991) gives an account of the use of 'victim support groups' using role-play and other activities in weekly groupwork sessions to develop children's social and friendship skills, self-esteem, assertiveness and ability to deal with conflict. The information about the evaluation of the approach in the original paper is somewhat sketchy, but Sharp and Cowie (1994) note that the children involved in Arora's study made gains in self-esteem, were judged to be more assertive in the classroom, and were less likely to be bullied, and they report similar outcomes from the Sheffield Project. Frederickson (1991) describes a related approach which focuses on social problem-solving. Thacker and Feest (1991) also report that interviews with 20 children one year after groupwork sessions ended revealed that the participants were more confident and had more effective social and conversational skills, and as a result were better able to talk about their problems and to listen to those of other people.

Solution-focused brief therapy (de Shazer, 1985) may also be appropriate for use with victims, but the caveat regarding the long-term effectiveness of the approach remains. However, at a more basic level, Olweus (1993) reports that victims can increase their self-esteem and popularity with their classmates merely by being given the opportunity to perform a useful activity.

Joint work with bullies and victims

The intervention approaches discussed so far have focused on dealing with bullies and victims separately. However, there are additional methods, all of which involve group-based problem-solving which can be used with joint groups of bullies and victims.

The 'Common Concern Method' for the treatment of group bullying

The 'Common Concern Method' (Pikas, 1989) is designed to tackle the problems of group bullying or 'mobbing' and is a development of an earlier technique, the 'Method of Shared Concern'. It involves a series of three stages of talks which must occur in a precise sequence: firstly, individual talks with each of the bullies; then an individual talk with the victim (suggestions are provided for dealing with the particular problems of provocative victims); and then either further talks with the bullies or a meeting with all of the bullies together with the victim. The aim of the process is to create a 'common feeling of concern' amongst the bullies by the use of non-threatening conflict resolution strategies in the talks and to foster a commitment to identify solutions to the problems of bullying. Pikas reports that case studies here show the technique to be effective (although no data is presented in the 1989 chapter) but also emphasises the considerable amount of training necessary for teachers to be able to use it. Smith *et al.* (1994) report that a follow-up study of the Method of Shared Concern involving thirty pupils and six teachers indicates that it is a useful technique in the short term, but that more enduring change may require the employment of additional interventions.

The 'No Blame' approach

The 'No Blame' approach (Maines and Robinson, 1991) also centres on establishing communication between victims, bullies and those who collude, by means of group meetings designed to allow the participants to express feelings. The victim's problem is explained to the group without blame being attributed and members are invited to use a problem-solving approach to suggest ways in which the problem might be resolved. Suggestions are collated and arrangements made to discuss developments individually with each member of the group after a week. As in the solution-focused approach (de Shazer, 1985) the adult mediator has the expectation that the bullies will act to solve the victim's problem.

The technique is similar to Pikas', although Maines and Robinson note that it is important to speak first to the victim, and to see the bullies initially in the group to facilitate the effects of peer pressure on change, a process which is also aided by emphasising the emotional distress experienced by the victim. The approach has not been formally evaluated, although case study data based on comments from teachers, parents and pupils are encouraging.

As a concluding comment, it should be noted that much of the research literature is concerned with the problems of the bullying which results from the actions of aggressive bullies, usually male, who engage in direct bullying. More research is needed to explore the efficacy of intervention approaches with female bullies, and those who engage in indirect bullying.

Class, school and community approaches

There has been little formal evaluation of the effectiveness of specific intervention at the class level, but examples of strategies reported in the literature include:

- checking on the bully or victim's relationships with their classmates and where necessary facilitating integration into the group (Besag, 1989)
- checking the educational attainment of the pupils involved in bullying and responding to any learning difficulties (Whitney *et al.*, 1994b; Mooney and Smith, 1995)

- asking a classmate or older pupil to monitor a victim's progress to provide information about social interactions and incidents of bullying, together with companionship and some measure of defence against further victimisation (Besag, 1989)
- ensuring that classroom supervision and seating arrangements do not contribute to bullying problems (Besag, 1989)

Within the school community there has been little formal evaluation of the effectiveness of measures when targeted on individual children, but examples of strategies include:

- keeping accurate records of incidents of bullying and how it was dealt with (Jones, 1991)
- monitoring supervision in areas of the school where specific incidents of bullying have been reported by the victim (e.g. in the playground, corridors, changing rooms, etc.) (Besag, 1991)

At the level of the wider community, possible strategies include:

- informing the parents of children involved in bullying either as perpetrator or victim and seeking their cooperation and involvement to ensure a consistent response to the difficulties and to encourage independence as well as caring empathetic relationships in the home (Besag, 1989; Pearce, 1991; Pepler *et al.*, 1993)
- seeking support for vulnerable pupils from the community as a whole (e.g. from youth clubs and other organisations for young people) (Tattum, 1993b)

Thus far we have considered reactive approaches to managing the problems of bullying. But such responses are dependent upon incidents being reported by the children, and as we have seen, this can be problematic given the secretive nature of bullying. In the next section we consider preventative strategies designed to reduce the prevalence of bullying throughout the school and their implications for school organisation and ethos.

THE PREVENTION OF BULLYING IN SCHOOLS

As Johnstone *et al.*, (1992) note, it is possible to use strategies proactively to respond to the problems of the individual pupils involved in bullying. For example, schools can review the nature of the support available to pupils and can prepare contingency plans for dealing with victims and bullies based upon the approaches discussed above.

Examples of preventative strategies at the class level include:

- *Encouraging an ethos of 'telling'* The importance of introducing procedures to encourage pupils to report bullying to teachers or parents is highlighted by Jones (1991) and Mellor (1991). However, this involves more than empowering victims to talk about their problems with their teachers, providing 'post boxes' for information from pupils to be passed on anonymously and encouraging teachers and peers to listen. As Cowie and Sharp (1994) point out, it also means engaging the much larger number of uninvolved 'bystanders'. They note that such pupils offer tacit support to bullies by ignoring the problems or remaining silent and suggest further that the often considerable between-class differences observed in the prevalence of bullying in schools may reflect an underlying class 'ethos' with regard to either passive or active support of bullying. An ethos which reinforces the view that bullying is unacceptable may encourage 'telling' and counter the 'bystander effect', and Cowie and Sharp argue that this can be developed by encouraging the values of cooperation and tolerance through the curriculum, citing evidence from work with children in multi-ethnic primary classrooms.

- *Using the curriculum* Smith and Sharp (1993) note that the curriculum can be used in two ways to tackle the problems of bullying: both to raise levels of 'awareness' and provide pupils with insight; and to facilitate behavioural change by means of drama and role play (Gobey, 1991), literature (Herbert, 1989) and personal and social education (Herbert, 1993).

Evaluation of such approaches has tended to involve case studies, with more emphasis upon the process (in terms of insight and awareness) than upon outcomes. However, Cowie and Sharp provide a review of the studies carried out as part of the DfE Sheffield Anti-Bullying Project and conclude that the two most effective approaches were 'Quality Circles', a cooperative group problem-solving approach applied to bullying behaviour (used in primary schools) which encouraged children to become more reflective and analytic, and a story about racial harassment, *The Heartstone Odyssey*, (used in primary schools with associated groupwork activities, role play, drama and discussions over two terms), which potentially facilitates high rates of disclosure of bullying and marked reductions in reports of being bullied.

Curricular approaches thus appear to provide a means of changing not only attitudes but perhaps also behaviour. While more research is required in this area, it is useful in the interim to note Cowie and Sharp's conclusion that the extent to which a curricular approach has an effect upon actual behaviour appears to be a function of the degree of group interaction and of the time involved. The use of 'one-off' videos or workshop activities is unlikely to result in any lasting changes.

- *Class rules* Olweus (1993) draws attention to the importance of introducing simple, clearly-expressed 'class rules' regarding bullying and of weekly 'class meetings' using literature, role play and videos to promote discussion. He reports that the classes in Norway which had the greatest reductions in bullying following a multi-level intervention programme were those which had implemented this approach, which again appears to exemplify the principle that effective change is likely to occur following sustained, group activities involving cooperation and discussion.

At the level of the school as a whole, there is a consensus that schools should attempt to determine the scale of the problem and to identify where bullying tends to occur (Johnstone *et al.*, 1992; Olweus, 1993; Smith and Sharp, 1994a). As we saw in the previous chapter, this can be done by means of anonymous self-report questionnaires which provide a valid measure of the prevalence of bullying, although there are still some question-marks regarding test–retest reliability. Pupils can also be encouraged to write about their lives in school and their responses used to locate bullying 'hot spots'.

- *Improving supervision* Following the above, it may be desirable to increase adult supervision of the places where bullying tends to occur in the school (e.g. playgrounds, corridors, lavatories, etc.) (Besag, 1989) and to make 'spot checks'.

  This has led to a number of interesting initiatives which indicate that playground bullying can be significantly reduced by the provision of training for the supervisors, raising their status within the school, tracking levels of bullying in the playground, responding promptly to problems using agreed sanctions, and by the provision of games and play equipment to help foster social skills and cooperative activity (Blatchford, 1993; Boulton, 1994; MacKay and Briggs, 1994).
- *School rules* The involvement of a range of teaching and non-teaching staff in supervision duties also highlights the need for school managers to coordinate and monitor the school's disciplinary policy to ensure coherent, consistent responses to the problems (Tattum, 1993b).
- *Procedures for transition from primary to secondary and for integrating a new pupil* The point of transfer from home to primary school or from primary to secondary school can be a time of anxiety for pupils. Tattum (1993b) also provides examples of the concerns reported by pupils and notes the need for schools to develop induction programmes to prepare pupils prior to the transfer and to help them adjust after. Such programmes can also be used to help integrate new pupils who transfer into the school at other times.
- *Staff development and training* The importance of providing training for playground supervisors so that they can identify incidents of bullying and deal with them appropriately was noted above (Boulton, 1994). Munn (1993) also makes a case for involving the wide range of

non-teaching staff (e.g. auxiliaries, office staff, caretaking staff, bus drivers, etc.). Many of the strategies discussed thus far have implications for training but it is worth noting that training designed merely to raise awareness is unlikely to change teachers' behaviour. As Joyce and Showers (1988) note, effective staff development has to contain not only theory and illustrative examples but also practice, feedback and opportunities for 'coaching'. Evidence from the DfE Sheffield Anti-Bullying Project bears this out: the greatest reductions in bullying behaviour in primary schools were associated with the highest levels of staff involvement and engagement in determining their school's anti-bullying policy.

- *Communication with all pupils and staff* Good communication with pupils and staff is an important aspect of preventing bullying. It is necessary, firstly, to raise awareness about the problems; secondly, to promote discussion and consultation to set an agenda for dealing with bullying; and thirdly, to ensure that all staff and pupils are aware of school rules, policies and ethos. Olweus (1993) suggests that schools should organise a 'conference' involving all staff and representatives from parents, pupils, external agencies and school governors to discuss the problems and move towards effective action. He also recommends regular small-group meetings for teachers as a forum for sharing experience and ideas on dealing with bullying, which may serve as a useful vehicle for staff development.

Bullying is not only a problem for schools but for the community as a whole. We have discussed the involvement of parents of bullies and victims in dealing with bullying, but parents also have a part to play in shaping the school's perception of what should be considered as bullying behaviour, and should be consulted about policy in this area. Parents also need to know what to do if they suspect their child is being bullied in school (see Mellor, 1993; Munn, 1993).

Attitudes in the local community towards bullying may also influence children's views and publicising anti-bullying initiatives more widely in the local area may provide additional support for a school. The involvement of local personalities or representatives from business may serve to attract people to meetings and thus increase awareness of the problems as a precursor to action.

External support agencies such as educational psychology services and social services departments may also be able to provide expertise and practical help in areas such as groupwork, counselling, and design and analysis of surveys.

EVIDENCE FOR THE EFFECTIVENESS OF WHOLE-SCHOOL APPROACHES TO INTERVENTION

Given the complexity of the nature of bullying and of schools as organisations there has been great interest in 'whole school' approaches: multi-level responses combining elements of both management and prevention (see Johnstone *et al.*, 1992; Olweus, 1993; Tattum, 1993a; DfE, (1994). Such approaches are generally summarised in the form of a whole-school anti-bullying policy, which is a written statement of the school's ethos with regard to bullying (e.g. 'fostering cooperation and respect for others'), its aims (e.g. 'reducing the levels of bullying behaviours') and the strategies and procedures to be used to achieve these (DfE, 1994).

A whole-school policy provides a means of coordinating specific approaches at the different levels within the school system and unsurprisingly has been a component of a number of studies evaluating the effectiveness of intervention. Table 11.1 summarises the outcomes from four large-scale studies.

Olweus (1991; 1994) evaluated the effectiveness of a 20-month whole-school programme across 42 schools. The programme incorporated strategies at individual, class and school levels involving school staff, pupils, parents and psychologists (see also Olweus, 1993 for details). The strategies were derived from Olweus' research into aggressive behaviour and were designed to tackle bullying, after an initial survey of its prevalence, by means of: positive and active involvement by adults; explicit rules setting limits for unacceptable behaviour; discussion of bullying in class using video materials and role play; 'non-physical' sanctions; monitoring and improved surveillance of behaviour, particularly in the playground; discussions with bullies and victims; and parental involvement.

The effectiveness of the intervention was determined by means of time-lagged comparisons between large age-equivalent groups using a 'cohort sequential' design. This involves comparing the prevalence of bullies and victims among 12-year-olds at the start of the programme, for example, with the prevalence among different 12-year-olds after the programme.

Olweus' key findings (from anonymous pupil self-report questionnaires administered 20 months after the start of the programme) were the halving of rates of both direct and indirect bullying 'now and then' or more frequently for both boys and girls, bullies and victims; a reduction in truancy and anti-social behaviour generally; and increases in pupil levels of satisfaction with school. He also noted that the effects of intervention were more marked after 20 months than after one year.

Roland (1989) evaluated the success of the original nationwide anti-bullying campaign in Norway by examining levels of bullying in 37 schools three years after the campaign. The original programme involved surveying the prevalence of bullying, distributing a booklet containing

Table 11.1 Summary of findings from published intervention studies

Study	No. in sample	Intervention period	Outcomes
Olweus (1991; 1994)	2,500 pupils aged 11–14 years in 112 classes in 42 schools in Norway	20 months	Pupil self-report questionnaires showed reductions of around 50% in bullying behaviour 'now and then' or more frequently in school
Roland (1989; 1993)	7,000 pupils aged 8–15 years in 37 schools in Norway	3 years: but no specific input from project team	Pupil self-report questionnaires revealed a slight rise in bullying behaviour in the case of males (e.g. from 3.6% to 5.2% in the case of victims and from 4.1% to 5.1% for bullies). No change in the prevalence of bullying behaviour among girls which remained below 2%
Pepler *et al.* (1993)	898 pupils aged 11–14 years in 4 schools in Toronto	7 months	Self-report questionnaire data revealed no change in the number of pupils bullied 'more than once or twice' but a reduction in the number of pupils 'bullied in the last 5 days' (from 13% to 9%) and a similar fall in the number of pupils socially excluded by their peers
Whitney, *et al.* (1994a)	6,468 pupils aged 8–16 years in 23 schools (16 primaries and 7 secondaries). Data also from 1,842 pupils in 4 comparison (non-intervention) schools (1 primary and 3 secondaries)	21 months (i.e. from the first meetings to formulate whole-school policies)	Self-report questionnaire data showed a drop of 17% in bullying behaviour in primary schools but a 2% rise in bullying behaviour in secondaries. Pupil questionnaires revealed a reduction of 46% in bullying in the playground in primaries. Significant associations between staff involvement in policy development and (a) decreases in bullying in the case of primary schools and (b) the likelihood of disclosing bullying to a teacher in the secondaries

advice on tackling bullying and a video to schools with pupils aged between 8 and 16 years, and requiring the schools to send out a folder of advice to parents.

Roland's results, showing slight overall increases of 1–2 per cent in bullying rates for boys appear disappointing at first sight. But the results are entirely predictable: the schools did not receive any additional intervention apart from the provision of the materials above, and most did not discuss the policy issues or use the materials with pupils. In cases where they did, there were reports of reductions in bullying. But in the main, merely raising awareness and providing information about bullying is not enough to ensure change.

However, one further major difference between the two Norwegian studies should be noted: Roland used a stricter criterion for bullying (of 'once a week or more') than Olweus ('now and then' or more frequently). While this focused Roland's enquiry upon the most serious, persistent bullying it had the disadvantage of lowering the base rates of bullying, which may have resulted in a less sensitive indicator of change (see Farrington, 1993).

Data from the 'Toronto Bullying Survey' (Pepler et al., 1993) reveals no change in the number of pupils bullied 'more than once or twice' but a reduction in the number of pupils 'bullied in the last 5 days' (from 13 per cent to 9 per cent) and a similar fall in the number of pupils socially excluded by their peers, in response to a whole-school anti-bullying programme. The criterion of being 'bullied in the last five days' is problematic, as it may include 'one-off' incidents. However, although the overall results may be disappointing when compared with Olweus', the intervention was carried out over only seven months, which may be too short a time for such school-based initiatives to 'bed in'.

Whitney et al. (1994a) report the findings from the 23 schools in Sheffield who took part in the Sheffield Anti-Bullying Project together with data from four non-intervention schools. The project consisted of a 'Core' intervention, a whole-school policy, to which individual schools were able to add optional interventions including: curriculum-based approaches (video and drama, The Heartstone Odyssey, and Quality Circles), direct work with bullies and victims (assertiveness training, Pikas' 'Method of Shared Concern', bully courts and peer counselling) and playground initiatives (e.g. training for play supervisors, and landscaping playgrounds). The intervention period was around 21 months and outcomes were measured by means of pre- and post-intervention anonymous pupil self-report surveys, interviews with teachers, pupils and other staff, and interim monitoring of the optional interventions selected by the school. Comparisons were made between the pre- and post-test scores for schools, with adjustment to ensure comparability.

The results revealed an overall decrease of around 17 per cent in reports of bullying behaviour in participating primary schools but a slight (non-significant) increase in secondary schools. The *number* of pupils involved in incidents of bullying as bullies or victims did not change significantly as a result of intervention, but the *frequency* of reported incidents of bullying did fall significantly: there was a reduction in the frequency of bullying reported by victims (by 14 per cent in the primary schools and by 7 per cent in the secondaries) and by bullies (by around 12 per cent in both primaries and secondaries). In addition, interim monitoring also revealed a fall of 46 per cent in the frequency of bullying in the playground in primary schools.

DISCUSSION

As we saw in the previous chapter, bullying can have long-term effects for both victims and perpetrators. However, the results reviewed here demonstrate that despite considerable variation between studies it is possible to reduce levels of bullying in schools. But it should be noted that the actual number of pupils involved in bullying may be largely unaffected by intervention, as in the Sheffield study. This implies that bullying may never be completely eradicated from schools and may help to shape realistic expectations of successful outcomes.

The gains reported by the Sheffield study were not as impressive as those reported by Olweus, but there are a number of points which should be borne in mind particularly when considering the relative effectiveness of intervention in primary and secondary schools. Firstly, the lower overall base-rate of bullying amongst secondary school pupils makes change harder to detect, even when less conservative criteria such as being bullied 'this term', or 'now and then' are used. Secondly, there were only seven secondary schools in the Sheffield sample, with particularly marked between-school differences which complicated the interpretation of the results. Thirdly, there are problems in trying to identify which of the optional interventions selected by individual schools were most suitable for the primary or secondary sectors. Fourthly, secondary schools are more complex organisations than primary schools and it may be more difficult to implement policies and to effect change at a whole-school level. And fifthly, the results from the Sheffield study also reveal that 30 per cent of secondary pupils indicated that they would report bullying to a teacher compared with only 7 per cent in the primaries. This suggests that the intervention encouraged the development of a 'telling ethos' in secondary schools, which in itself is a positive outcome, but one which also raises the question of whether the less dramatic reductions in reports of bullying in secondaries were in part the result of an increased likelihood of reporting bullying following intervention. Clearly, more longitudinal research studies are necessary to clarify this issue.

CONCLUSION

It is possible to draw the following conclusions from the overall pattern of results:

1 significant reductions in bullying can be achieved by means of a whole-school approach but merely providing schools with information is unlikely to achieve change;
2 schools vary in the extent to which they can commit themselves to a whole-school approach;
3 the duration of the intervention is important: change is a gradual process and the benefits may only become apparent after two years, particularly given the indirect nature of the outcome measures used;
4 the reductions in bullying in the Sheffield study were much less marked than in Olweus' (although there are some differences between schools and society in the two countries which may have an effect upon outcomes – see Tattum, 1993b);
5 intervention in the Sheffield study appeared to be more successful in the primary schools, but pupils in secondaries were more likely to report incidents to their teachers in schools where there was a high level of staff involvement in both developing a whole-school policy and in introducing the optional interventions, which may reflect the emergence of a 'telling ethos';
6 further studies are needed to identify the most effective elements of a whole-school approach (see Farrington, 1993); but there is also a need for care in selecting appropriate outcome measures and for realistic expectations about what constitutes a successful outcome.

In the past, schools may have been reluctant to address the problems of bullying because of uncertainty about the outcomes and the implications for staff development and resourcing (Thompson and Smith (1991). However, the results from large-scale studies in the UK and Scandinavia confirm that a successful whole-school approach to the management and prevention of bullying with the following elements may lead to the development of a more positive ethos, with wide-ranging benefits for those who bully and those who are bullied alike:

• an anti-bullying policy which communicates concern about bullying and emphasises that it will not be tolerated. The policy should also stress a 'telling ethos' and an ethos of mutual respect and concern for others. It should be widely publicised and deal with school rules, rewards and punishments, the monitoring and recording of bullying, procedures for supporting victims and dealing with bullies, and procedures for new entrants. Staff, pupils and parents alike should be involved in its development to ensure joint ownership;
• surveys to establish the extent of the bullying problem. These can also

serve as a focus for discussion of intervention approaches;

- social skills training and approaches such as the 'Method of Common Concern' for individuals and groups involved in bullying;
- supervision in the playground together with training for the supervisors;
- cooperative groupwork activities in class focusing upon anti-bullying themes.

REFERENCES

Ahmad, Y., Whitney, I. and Smith, P. K. (1991) 'A survey service for schools on bully/victim problems', in P. K. Smith and D. A. Thompson (eds) *Practical Approaches to Bullying*, London: David Fulton.

Arora, T. (1991) 'The use of victim support groups', in P. K. Smith and D. A. Thompson (eds) *Practical Approaches to Bullying*, London: David Fulton.

Besag, V. (1989) *Bullies and Victims in Schools: A Guide to Understanding and Management*, Buckingham: Open University Press.

—— (1991) 'The playground', in M. Elliott (ed.) *Bullying: A Practical Guide to Coping For Schools*, Harlow, Essex: Longman.

—— (1992) *We Don't Have Bullies Here*! V. Besag, 57 Manor House Road, Jesmond, Newcastle-upon-Tyne NE2 2LY.

Blatchford, P. (1993) 'Bullying in the playground', in D. Tattum (ed.) *Understanding and Managing Bullying*, Oxford: Heinemann Educational.

Boulton, M. (1994) 'Preventing bullying in the playground', in P. K. Smith and S. Sharp (eds) *School Bullying: Insights and Perspectives*, London: Routledge.

Brier, J. and Ahmad, Y. (1991) 'Developing a school court as a means of addressing bullying in schools', in P. K. Smith and D. A. Thompson (eds) *Practical Approaches to Bullying*, London: David Fulton.

Byrne, B. (1994) *Coping with Bullying in Schools*, London: Cassell.

Chazan, M. (1989) 'Bullying in the infant school', in D. P. Tattum and D. A. Lane (eds) *Bullying in Schools*, Stoke-on-Trent: Trentham Books.

Coie, J. D., Underwood, M. and Lochman, J. E. (1991) 'Programmatic intervention with aggressive children in the school setting', in D. J. Pepler and K. H. Rubin (eds) *The Development and Treatment of Childhood Aggression*, Hillsdale, New Jersey: Lawrence Erlbaum Associates.

Cowie, H. and Sharp, S. (1994) 'Tackling bullying through the curriculum', in P. K. Smith and S. Sharp (eds) *School Bullying: Insights and Perspectives*, London: Routledge.

Department for Education (1994) *Bullying: Don't Suffer in Silence. An Anti-bullying Pack for Schools*, London: HMSO.

Department of Education and Science (1989) *Discipline in Schools* (The Elton Report), London: HMSO.

de Shazer, S. (1985) *Keys to Solution in Brief Therapy*, Norton: New York.

Drouet, D. (1993) 'Adolescent female bullying and sexual harassment', in D. Tattum (ed.) *Understanding and Managing Bullying*, Oxford: Heinemann Educational.

Elliott, M. (1986) 'KIDSCAPE Primary Kit', London: Kidscape.

—— (1989) 'Bullying – harmless fun or murder', in E. Munthe and E. Roland (eds) *Bullying: An International Perspective*, London: David Fulton.

—— (1991a) 'Bullies, victims, signs, solutions', in M. Elliott (ed.) *Bullying: A Practical Guide to Coping for Schools*, Harlow, Essex: Longman.

—— (1991b) *Bullying: A Practical Guide to Coping for Schools*, Harlow, Essex: Longman.

—— (1991c) 'Bully "courts"', in M. Elliott (ed.) *Bullying: A Practical Guide to Coping for Schools*, Harlow, Essex: Longman.

Farrington, D. P. (1993) 'Understanding and preventing bullying', in M. Tonry (ed.) *Crime and Justice: A Review of Research Vol. 17*, Chicago: The University of Chicago Press.

Foster, P. and Thompson, D. (1991) 'Bullying: towards a non-violent sanctions policy', in P. K. Smith and D. Thompson (eds) *Practical Approaches to Bullying*, London: David Fulton.

Frederickson, N. (1991) 'Children can be so cruel: helping the rejected child', in G. Lindsay and A. Miller (eds) *Psychological Services for Primary Schools*, Harlow, Essex: Longman.

Frost, L. (1991) 'A primary school approach – what can be done about the bully?' in M. Elliott (ed.) *Bullying: A Practical Guide to Coping for Schools*, Harlow, Essex: Longman.

Gillborn, D. (1993) 'Racial violence and bullying', in D. Tattum (ed.) *Understanding and Managing Bullying*, Oxford: Heinemann Educational.

Gobey, F. (1991) 'A practical approach through drama and workshops', in P. K. Smith and D. A. Thompson (eds) *Practical Approaches to Bullying*, London: David Fulton.

Herbert, G. (1989) 'A whole curriculum approach to bullying', in D. P. Tattum and D. A. Lane (eds) *Bullying in Schools*, Stoke-on-Trent: Trentham Books.

—— (1993) 'Changing children's attitudes through the curriculum', in D. Tattum (ed.) *Understanding and Managing Bullying*, Oxford: Heinemann Educational Books.

Higgins, C. (1994) 'Improving the school ground environment as an anti-bullying intervention', in P. K. Smith and S. Sharp (eds) *School Bullying: Insights and Perspectives*, London: Routledge.

Johnstone, M., Munn, P. and Edwards, L. (1992) *Action against Bullying: A Support Pack for Schools*, Edinburgh: The Scottish Council for Research in Education.

Jones, E. (1991) 'Practical considerations in dealing with bullying – in secondary school', in M. Elliott (ed.) *Bullying: A Practical Guide to Coping for Schools*, Harlow, Essex: Longman.

Joyce, B. and Showers, B. (1988) *Student Achievement through Staff Development*. Longman: New York.

La Fontaine, J. (1991) *Bullying: The Child's View*, London: Calouste Gulbenkian Foundation.

Laslett, R. (1982) 'A children's court for bullies', *Special Education*, 9: 9–11.

Lowenstein, L. F. (1991) 'The study, diagnosis and treatment of bullying in a therapeutic community, in M. Elliott (ed.) *Bullying: A Practical Guide to Coping for Schools*, Harlow, Essex: Longman.

MacKay, T. and Briggs, S. (1994) '"Fair Play": the primary school playground', *Educational Psychology in Scotland*, 2: 24–9.

Maines, B. and Robinson, G. (1991) 'Don't beat the bullies!', *Educational Psychology in Practice*, 7, 3: 168–72.

McLean, A. (1994) *Promoting Positive Relationships: Bullyproofing Our School*, Glasgow: Strathclyde Regional Council, Department of Education.

Mellor, A. (1990) *Bullying in Scottish Secondary Schools*, SCRE Spotlights Number 23, Edinburgh: The Scottish Council for Research in Education.

—— (1991) 'Helping victims', in M. Elliott (ed.) *Bullying: A Practical Guide to Coping for Schools*, Harlow, Essex: Longman.

—— (1993) *Bullying and How to Fight It: A Guide for Families*, Edinburgh: The Scottish Council for Research in Education.

Mooney, S. and Smith, P. K. (1995) 'Bullying and the child who stammers', *British Journal of Special Education*, 2, 1: 24–7.

Mortimore, P., Sammons, P., Ecob, R. and Stoll, L. (1988) *School Matters: The Junior Years*, London: Open Books.

Munn, P. (1993) *Supporting Schools against Bullying: The Second SCRE Anti-bullying Pack*, Edinburgh: The Scottish Council for Research in Education.

Munthe, E. (1989) 'Bullying in Scandinavia', in E. Roland and E. Munthe (eds) *Bullying: An International Perspective*, London: David Fulton.

Munthe, E. and Roland, E. (eds) (1989) *Bullying: An International Perspective*, London: David Fulton.

Olweus, D. (1984) 'Aggressors and their victims: bullying at school', in N. Frude and H. Gault (eds) *Disruptive Behaviour in Schools*, Chichester: John Wiley and Sons.

—— (1991) 'Bully / victim problems among schoolchildren: basic facts and effects of a school based intervention program', in D. J. Pepler and K. H. Rubin (eds) *The Development and Treatment of Childhood Aggression*, Hillsdale, New Jersey: Lawrence Erlbaum Associates.

—— (1993) *Bullying at School: What We Know and What We Can Do*, Oxford: Blackwell.

—— (1994) 'Bullying at school: basic facts and effects of a school based intervention program', *Journal of Child Psychology and Psychiatry*, 35, 7: 1171–90.

Pearce, J. (1991) 'What can be done about the bully?', in M. Elliott (ed.) *Bullying: A Practical Guide to Coping for Schools*, Harlow, Essex: Longman.

Pepler, D., Craig., W., Ziegler, S. and Charach, A. (1993) 'A school-based anti-bullying intervention: preliminary evaluation', in D. Tattum (ed.) *Understanding and managing bullying*, Oxford: Heinemann Educational Books.

Pikas, A. (1989) 'The Common Concern Method for the treatment of mobbing', in E. Munthe and E. Roland (eds) *Bullying: An International Perspective*, London: David Fulton.

Priest, S. (1989) 'Some practical approaches to bullying', in E. Roland and E. Munthe (eds) *Bullying: An International Perspective*, London: David Fulton.

Roland, E. (1989) 'Bullying: the Scandinavian research tradition', in D. P. Tattum and D. A. Lane (eds) *Bullying in Schools*, Stoke-on-Trent: Trentham Books.

—— (1993) 'Bullying: a developing tradition of research and management', in D. Tattum (ed.) *Understanding and Managing Bullying*, Oxford: Heinemann Educational.

Rutter, M., Maughan, B., Mortimore, P. and Ouston, J. (1979) *Fifteen Thousand Hours: Secondary Schools and their Effects on Children*, London: Open Books.

Sharp, S. and Cowie, H. (1994) 'Empowering pupils to take positive action against bullying', in P. K. Smith and S. Sharp (eds) *School Bullying: Insights and Perspectives*, London: Routledge.

Sharp, S. and Smith, P. K. (1994) (eds) *Tackling Bullying in Your Schools: A Practical Handbook for Teachers*, London: Routledge.

Sharp, S. and Thompson, D. (1994) 'The role of whole-school policies in tackling bullying behaviour in schools', in P. K. Smith and S. Sharp (eds) *School Bullying: Insights and Perspectives*, London: Routledge.

Skinner, A. (1992) *Bullying: An Annotated Bibliography of Literature and Resources*, Leicester: Youth Work Press.

Smith, P. K. and Sharp, S. (1993) 'Tackling bullying: the Sheffield Project', in D. Tattum (ed.) *Understanding and Managing Bullying*, Oxford: Heinemann Educational Books.

Smith, P. K. and Sharp, S. (1994a) (eds) *School Bullying: Insights and Perspectives*, London: Routledge.

Smith, P. K. and Sharp, S. (1994b) 'The problem of school bullying', in P. K. Smith and S. Sharp (eds) *School Bullying: Insights and Perspectives*, London: Routledge.

Smith, P. K., Cowie, H. and Sharp, S. (1994c) 'Working directly with pupils involved in bullying situations', in P. K. Smith and S. Sharp (eds) *School Bullying: Insights and Perspectives*, London: Routledge.

Smith, P. K. and Thompson, D. (1991) (eds) *Practical Approaches to Bullying*, London: David Fulton.

Stephenson, P. and Smith, D. (1989) 'Bullying in the junior school', in D. P. Tattum and D. A. Lane (eds) *Bullying in Schools*, Stoke-on-Trent: Trentham Books.

Tattum, D. (1993a) (ed.) *Understanding and Managing Bullying*, Oxford: Heinemann Educational Books.

—— (1993b) 'Short, medium and long-term management strategies', in D. Tattum (ed.) *Understanding and Managing Bullying*, Oxford: Heinemann Educational Books.

Tattum, D. P. and Herbert, G. (1990) *Bullying – A Positive Response*, Faculty of Education, South Glamorgan Institute of Higher Education, Cardiff.

Tattum, D. and Herbert, G. (1993) (eds) *Countering Bullying: Initiatives by Schools and Local Authorities*, Stoke-on-Trent: Trentham Books.

Tattum, D. P. and Lane, D. A. (1989) (eds) *Bullying in Schools*, Stoke-on-Trent: Trentham Books.

Tattum, D., Tattum, E. and Herbert, G. (1993) *Cycle of Violence*, Cardiff: Drake Educational Associates.

Thacker, J. and Feest, G. (1991) 'Groupwork in the primary school', in G. Lindsay and A. Mills (eds) *Psychological Services for Primary Schools*, Harlow, Essex: Longman.

Thompson, D. and Smith, P. K. (1991) 'Effective action against bullying – the key problems', in P. K. Smith and D. Thompson (1991) (eds) *Practical Approaches to Bullying*, London: David Fulton.

Topping, K. (1983) *Educational Systems for Disruptive Adolescents*, London: Croom Helm.

Whitney, I. and Smith, P. K. (1993) 'A survey of the nature and extent of bullying in junior, middle and secondary schools', *Educational Research*, 35, 1: 3–25.

Whitney, I., Rivers, I., Smith, P. K. and Sharp, S. (1994a) 'The Sheffield Project: methodology and findings', in P. K. Smith and S. Sharp (eds) *School Bullying: Insights and Perspectives*, London: Routledge.

Whitney, I., Smith, P. K. and Thompson, D. (1994b) 'Bullying and children with special educational needs', in P. K. Smith and S. Sharp (eds) *School Bullying: Insights and Perspectives*, London: Routledge.

Yates, C. and Smith, P. K. (1989) 'Bullying in two English comprehensive schools', in E. Roland and E. Munthe (eds) *Bullying: An International Perspective*, London: David Fulton.

Chapter 12

Drug abuse: what's your poison?

John B. Davies

Throughout history, and in all parts of the world, human beings have shown a predilection for changing their states of consciousness by self-administering substances that alter the biochemistry of their brains. In most cases, the basic motivation is pleasure; on other occasions, the motivation may be less hedonistic: substances that ease the pain of physical or social trauma; or at a less exotic level, reduce stress or increase concentration. The range of substances used for these purposes is large, and before the advent of world travel, bore a closer relationship to local circumstances of climate and soil than to any agreed legal classifications of drugs. By and large, people used what was locally available; and by and large they learned to live with both the positive and negative consequences of using these substances. Even today, despite ease of travel, there are interesting deviations from what we in the West tend to view as 'normal'. Alcohol, a substance we use widely, whilst accepting that some individuals get into trouble through its use, is viewed in some Middle Eastern countries with the same dismay that we tend to view heroin use; and on the other hand in remote parts of Peru, workers on the land still chew coca leaves mixed with a little lime as they work in the fields, seemingly unaware of the fact that they are indulging in a drug widely viewed in the West as the most dangerous and addictive substance known to mankind.

World travel is now so easy, however, that regardless of where one lives one can find access to virtually the full menu of psychoactive substances without too much difficulty. This creates problems since substances now become available which are not part of indigenous culture, and which are not surrounded by sets of established mores and codes of social practice concerning their use. They are not part of the accepted 'ceremonial chemistry' (Szasz, 1985). At this point, logic flies out of the window, and the label 'drugs' is applied pejoratively to the new and strange substances coming from outside, simply because they are strange and new and therefore objects of fear. In the process they become imbued with properties and powers which they either do not have or which become much exaggerated.

This distinction ensures their inevitable absorption into the larger culture pattern is delayed, the activity becoming sidelined amongst minorities who are already viewed as deviant for other reasons ('drop-outs', 'the unemployed', 'blacks', etc). Their use thus remains 'abnormal', and the parent society battles to prevent the activity from spreading into the 'normal' population. Problems arise, however, when large numbers of (usually young) people start using these pharmacological exotica, since at that point large sections of the 'normal' population have to be reclassified as 'abnormal', and increasingly draconian measures are taken in the vain attempt to turn the clock back. Meanwhile the moral majority, whilst supporting these measures, continues with its coffee, tea, alcohol, nicotine and minor tranquilliser use, unaware of, or unwilling to accept, the fact that the only thing separating their own use of psychoactive substances from that of 'drug users' are certain accidents of history, geography and ease of travel.

COMPARING LICIT AND ILLICIT DRUG USE

Any chapter purporting to give a balanced view of the damage that drugs can cause both to people and to societies must begin by comparing licit and illicit drugs. In the UK at the present time something in excess of 90 per cent of the population drink alcohol from time to time, the majority experiencing few problems with this activity. On the other hand a smaller proportion drink alcohol in ways that are seriously damaging to health and well-being, and estimates suggest that alcohol may be a causal factor in some 15,000 deaths per annum. In fairness it should be pointed out that recent evidence suggests that a moderate level of alcohol consumption has a cardiovascular protective effect (Doll *et al.*, 1994). There is also strong evidence that the smoking habit is a major risk factor for heart disease and lung cancer, with smoking claimed to be causally involved in some 100,000 deaths per year in the UK (Royal College of Psychiatrists, 1987) and roughly four times that number in the USA (Report of the Surgeon General, 1989). Nonetheless the activities remain legal; alcohol consumption per capita continues to rise, and whilst smoking is currently on the decline, the nicotine habit is growing in certain sections of the population, notably teenage girls and younger women.

Without a doubt these two acceptable drugs are involved in more deaths than all the illicit drugs put together. Indeed the extent to which licit drug-related deaths exceed deaths due to the use of illicit drugs is quite remarkable. Home Office statistics suggest that deaths due to the use of illicit substances have run at the level of some 400 to 600 deaths per year for a number of years, though recent figures suggest this may have doubled in a short space of time. What is interesting, however, is the relative equanimity with which people contemplate the activities of smoking cigarettes and drinking alcohol, compared to the use of 'drugs' (i.e. non-approved ways of changing one's state of consciousness). Whilst we may be seriously concerned as parents if our offspring, particularly girls, show an increased tendency to smoke cigarettes or a predilection for the consumption of pints of beer, in some ways we feel that we are venturing into known territory – perhaps we don't like it, but we do not regard it as unnatural or abnormal. On the other hand, the use of illicit drugs by youngsters is seen by many people as a sign that things are seriously wrong either with the child involved, or his parents and peer group; a reaction far in excess of the response to discovering that a son or daughter has started to drink or smoke. Where illicit drugs are concerned the reaction involves fear and dismay.

In recent years surveys have been conducted seeking to discover the extent of use of illicit substances by young people. Whilst there are regional differences between the results of some of these studies, there is also a good deal of consensus. Studies carried out in London (Swadi, 1988), Manchester (Newcombe et al., 1994), Glasgow (Davies and Coggans, 1991) and Edinburgh (Plant et al., 1985) vary at the level of detail but confirm the general impression that the use of illicit drugs is no longer confined to a minority of 'sick children'. All these surveys suggest that between 25 and 35 per cent of young people of secondary school age (14 and above) have at least some experience of illicit drug use, with some figures being rather higher. For the majority of youngsters the drug involved is cannabis and the level of use is occasional. Nonetheless the studies also confirm the existence of smaller percentages of the teenage population who use drugs on a more regular basis, perhaps weekly or monthly, and who also perhaps venture into some of the more feared substances such as LSD or amphetamine (a class B drug from which is derived the class A drug ecstasy). Data collected by Swadi (1988) from a sample of London teenagers aged 11 to 16 years give a fairly typical picture (see Table 12.1).

In other words, drug use by young people is no longer sidelined: an abnormal exercise carried out by a small deviant minority. Instead, a sizeable proportion of youngsters, most of whom are perfectly normal and healthy, now have experience of at least the milder forms of illicit drug use. Similarly, in a survey of students at a Scottish university carried out in 1994, 44 per cent reported having used cannabis, 22 per cent LSD, 22 per cent amphetamines and 6 per cent ecstasy. Everyday use was reported by 9 per cent, and weekly use by 29 per cent of students (McAleese, 1994). In such circumstances it becomes reasonable to ask whether any policy aimed at stamping out this activity is likely to succeed. Have we simply not tried hard enough? Do we need stronger measures to eliminate this problem? Should we prosecute and punish half the teenage population of the country for smoking cannabis? Or is it

Table 12.1 Type of substance, frequency of use and gender of user

Substance	Gender	Only once/occasionally %	Weekly/daily %
Cannabis	M[a]	50	9
	F[b]	48	7
Solvents	M	42	4
	F	53	12
Stimulants	M	14	2
	F	13	3
Tranquillisers	M	11	0.8
	F	14	0.8
Cocaine	M	6	0.5
	F	9	5
Hallucinogens	M	10	1
	F	6	0.8
Heroin	M	4	3
	F	4	6

Source: Taken from Swadi, 1988

Notes: [a]n (male) = 377; [b]n (female) = 253

more sensible to concede that the horse has bolted and is long past the point at which sensible legal sanctions will get it back into the stable?

The response to illicit drug use

Increases in the use of illicit drugs by all sections of the population, both in the UK and elsewhere, have led to an increase in the concern shown by government, media and the population generally about the effects of drugs on society. Concern about this expansion in the use of what are still to many people largely unknown and misunderstood substances has been brought more sharply into focus by the disproportionate rise in the number of young people now apparently prepared to experiment with illicit drugs, and the growth in what is termed 'recreational drug use' by this age group in a variety of settings. The evidence tends to come from surveys conducted amongst samples of youngsters attending school, or via youth groups for the most part; and in the main the data show that long term health or social consequences are rare in this group. Even rarer are reports of use of the so-called 'hard' drugs such as heroin and cocaine amongst this age group. In our own Scottish study, (Coggans *et al.*, 1991) self-reported heroin use ran at the same rate as the use of 'astrolite', a fictitious drug invented specially for the survey. It is clear that for most youngsters the most acute danger lies in the possibility of arrest, prosecution and a criminal record, rather than risks to health or social functioning. It is also clear that the vast majority of these youngsters do not progress to become 'addicts'.

However, to the extent that such samples may selectively exclude those youngsters having the most severe problems, and who are therefore less likely to be at school or to attend organised youth groups, it may be argued that the current prevalence data underestimate the scale of the problem, or at least, that some of the most severe problem cases fall through the net. At a local level it is also possible to identify groups with more serious drug use careers, areas of inner cities where these figures may be considerably higher within a confined locality and areas where younger and sometimes very young children will be involved in the use of drugs. There is no doubt, therefore, on the basis of these studies, that the use of illicit drugs amongst young people has increased dramatically and shows no sign of abating; and that for small but significant numbers of users the outlook is far from reassuring.

Nonetheless, the images of mass youthful 'drug abuse' and 'teenage addicts' that haunt the media are generally inaccurate and do not reflect fairly on the behaviour of most of those involved. Prominence is given to those instances in which use of drugs by teenagers results in catastrophe both for a family and for the individual involved simply because, although such stories are not typical, they are newsworthy. 'Teenager takes drugs, has fun, and passes five A-levels' is not a headline that sells newspapers. At the time of writing, South Ayrshire in Scotland has become a focus for media attention following four drug related deaths at weekend raves held at venues on the Ayrshire coast. It appears that while the rave scene within Glasgow is perhaps subject to tighter controls, coachloads of youngsters leave the city centre at certain times of the week in order to attend raves some 30 miles away in the more rural parts of Ayrshire. Evidence shows that rave drugs are readily available on these coaches, and that 'drug pushing' (or to be more accurate, the sale of drugs to youngsters who actively want to buy them) begins almost as soon as the youngsters embark on their bus journey. There is great concern about the deaths amongst this group which are connected to the use of ecstasy, but which possibly involve other drugs and behaviours not yet documented. The picture therefore looks grave. In such a context the understandable reaction of many parents to the discovery that their offspring are involved in any way with this kind of activity and these kinds of dance drugs becomes a cause for family disruption, fear and an unqualified over-reaction, especially when local events conspire to produce lurid illustrations of the perils of drug use close to hand. However, without being blasé about the issues involved, it is reasonable to conclude that whilst the four deaths are tragic and require close investigation, four deaths from amongst a participating group numbering some tens of thousands within the region is not yet an epidemic, although it is clearly four deaths too many.

It is clear that drugs can and do kill. It is also clear, however, that an account of drug use which stresses the damage to health and the mortality rate without giving attention to the dynamics of the broader drug scene is in danger of creating a caricature of the drug use situation amongst young people. One can imagine, for example, the use of motor cars being portrayed as a highly dangerous and undesirable activity if one were to produce repeated media accounts focusing entirely on the numbers of people killed and maimed on the road but making no reference to the far larger number of people who successfully move from A to B with enjoyment and without trauma. It is possible to place the real hazard of drug use by youngsters in a broader context which makes both their behaviour more comprehensible and presents a less frightening picture. Whilst drug use is involved in a number of fatalities each year, the vast majority of people who use illicit drugs experience no long-term health or social consequences arising from that drug use. This is probably more true of young drug users than any other group. The data show that chronic or dependent long-term drug habits are rare in the teenage group. Furthermore, the attitude of teenagers who are themselves users of so-called 'recreational drugs' (cannabis, amphetamine/ecstasy, LSD) is very much in line with the attitudes of the older population when it comes to use of the more feared drugs (Parker and Measham, 1994). Whilst many teenagers view their own use of dance and rave drugs as in some sense 'all right', their view of the helpless junkie who uses heroin and cocaine tends to be as stereotyped and inaccurate as the views of the rest of the population. In a word, therefore, most youngsters using recreational drugs do not see themselves as belonging in any way to a 'junkie' or drug addict type of culture (Henderson et al., 1993). From a prevention point of view this set of attitudes may even be a good thing if it prevents movement from the dance and rave drugs to opiates.

DRUG USE AND CONTEXT

Central to most people's fear of illicit drugs is an inaccurate perception of the power that drugs wield. Despite massive research evidence to the contrary, the public perception of drug use is that the pharmacology of the drugs is sufficient to specify particular forms of behaviour. Thus, to use drugs is to fall under the power of drugs as part of an inexorable process. Freedom of decision is lost, drug-using behaviour becomes compelled by the pharmacology of the drug itself and various kinds of associated behaviours such as crime and prostitution inevitably follow. Even amongst pharmacologists, however, such a single factor type of determinism is not accepted. Data show that the precise impact that drug use has on an individual or on a society depends not merely on the drug in question but on a variety of other factors. These include the social circumstances of the people involved, the broader social networks and practices of the culture within which the family lives, and at an individual level the goals and aspirations of the persons who actually take the drugs themselves (Hawkins *et al.*, 1992). It is simply not the case that the drug predetermines the behaviour. In an analogous way, whilst there are heated debates about the supposed addictiveness of different substances, it remains the case that no substance exists which has the inherent capacity to cause addiction in all cases; and at the other extreme it must be conceded that there is no individual who cannot become dependent on a drug given certain social, economic and other circumstances. The state of addiction, therefore, arises as a consequence of a dialectic or interplay of factors involving individuals in particular social settings. The way that drug use manifests itself in any given situation depends on the type of lives available to or being led by the people in those circumstances and their drug of choice. This is true not merely of the so-called 'soft' drugs, but of drugs like heroin and cocaine also.

Until recently, most of the evidence on cocaine use has come from samples of people attending clinics, hospitals, and other agencies providing services for 'addicts'. The picture of cocaine use that emerges from such samples parallels the picture that would emerge if we based our views of 'typical alcohol use' entirely on samples drawn from Alcoholics Anonymous, councils on alcohol, and other agencies dealing with alcohol problems. However, recent community studies of cocaine use have revealed that most users of cocaine manage the habit successfully whilst a small percentage do not (Addiction Research, Special Issue: Cocaine in the Community, 1994). It is apparent that tales about cocaine such as 'I tried it once and I was hooked' do justice only to the smaller number of users who fail to manage the habit successfully; but no justice at all to the far larger numbers who do, but are not advertising the fact. This recent issue of *Addiction Research*, an international journal, was devoted entirely to this question, and revealed that most cocaine users in the community as a whole manage the habit in a controlled manner and do not become addicted. The data come from independent studies carried out in the USA, Canada, Scotland, the Netherlands and Australia, and show basically the same picture.

Despite the well documented fact that 'addiction' is as much a social as a pharmacological phenomenon, it is depressing to note that in the media and elsewhere the view of drugs as being the single determining factor with respect to the outcome of a drug use career continues to dominate.

The general picture, that most people who use drugs control the habit just as most of us control our alcohol consumption, whilst a smaller number fail to do so sometimes with catastrophic personal consequences, fails to impinge on the argument: the more damaging account continues to be preferred.

THE DRUG WARS OR 'LEARNING TO LIVE WITH IT'

In general terms there appear to be two broad philosophies with respect to dealing with the problems caused by illicit drug use. The more popular of these amongst the general adult population of the UK and many other countries, is to fight a 'war' on the drug problem. The aim of this policy is to create a drug-free society and the means by which this is attained consist of various types of police and judicial measures aimed at curtailing the activities of those who use and particularly who deal in illicit drugs. This so-called war on drugs is being fought in the UK, USA and a number of European countries, with the Netherlands standing out as being the one country which pursues a rather different policy. The second approach starts from the assumption that the war on drugs has already failed in spectacular fashion and in principle cannot succeed. A popular argument from this side draws an analogy with the era of prohibition in the United States. It is a matter of record that whilst some success might be claimed for this policy, it is also the case that alcohol use became surrounded by violence and gangsterism during that period. Certainly one could not claim that the era of prohibition succeeded in eradicating alcohol from American society. It follows that if drugs cannot be eradicated, alternative strategies have to be adopted to enable people to live in a society where drugs are in circulation whilst minimising the individual and collective harm that may arise from their misuse. There are several aspects to this argument but decriminalisation, and the philosophy of harm reduction (which will be discussed in the next chapter) are key components.

Can we win the drug wars?

Data are available on the number of people who have been prosecuted under current drug legislation and the sentences which were imposed over a period of some ten or fifteen years for those who were found guilty. One of the most focused studies in this area was carried out by Haw which examined data gathered from the Scottish Office and the Home Office. Using these data Haw was able to demonstrate that between 1980 and 1986, without any changes in the law as it stood, sentencing policy nonetheless changed markedly (Haw, 1989) as illustrated in Table 12.2. Effectively Haw's data show a process of 'criminalisation'; and it will be argued here that if such a process is possible without a change in the law then a process of decriminalisation may also be envisaged within the law as it stands.

Haw's data show a marked increase both in the number and severity of sentences handed down to people convicted of drug offences (mainly possession with intent to supply) over this period, with the year 1985–86 representing a high spot. In fairness it must be mentioned that the harshness of sentences has to some extent been reduced in recent years and that more pragmatic policies are being implemented in some areas, especially with respect to minor offences of possession with intent to supply. During the period 1980–86 Haw also demonstrated that sentences for class B drug offences, mainly cannabis, became virtually indistinguishable from sentences for trafficking in the 'harder' class A drugs, mainly heroin. This change in sentencing policy with respect to cannabis took place at a time when no comparable change was observed for a variety of offences involving theft, aggravated assault and other anti-social acts. There was also a drastic increase in the number of people being prosecuted to the extent that the high court time taken up with drug offences increased from a negligible amount (about 1 per cent) to 26 per cent over the time period. Taking Haw's data overall, therefore, we can see clear implications of the implementation of a tougher line as a response to a 'drug war' type of philosophy. Similar trends are observable in the United States, and in Europe the Netherlands is coming under increasing political pressure to take a tougher line (Leuw and Haen Marshall, 1994).

It is possible to compare this increase in drug war activity with statistics on the prevalence of drug use in the UK throughout that period. At the time of writing a variety of estimates of drug use amongst young people is available. As we have seen, whilst these vary according to locality, in general terms the data indicate that somewhere between 30

Table 12.2 Length of sentence for convicted drug offenders sentenced to custodial disposals in Scottish courts, 1980–86

Sentence length	1980	1981	1982	1983	1984	1985	1986
Up to 6 mths	27	28	64	65	129	139	152
> 6 mths–2 yrs	5	7	7	25	77	104	97
> 2 yrs–5 yrs	3	2	6	10	25	75	83
> 5 yrs	0	0	5	9	55	90	59
Unknown[a]	2	2	4	9	0	0	0

Source: Data adapted from Haw (1989)

Notes: Chi^2 = 125.56, $p < 0.001$, 18df; [a]unknown, excluded from analysis

and 45 per cent of young people have had some experience of illicit drug use (Swadi, 1988; Davies and Coggans, 1991; Plant *et al.*, 1985). This is a sizeable proportion of the youthful population, and though the data also suggest that this drug experience is extremely limited for most of the young people described by this statistic, nonetheless some form of drug use is within the experience of a sizeable minority, if not a majority, of the under-20 population. It remains only to add that the available data indicate that this present level of drug use is a substantial increase on earlier figures collected over the last ten years; and this steady increase in prevalence has also been accompanied by an increase in the number and variety of drugs available. In addition, drug seizures escalate both in value and size with each year that passes, probably indicating that more and more drugs are in circulation. It is worth considering also that the replacement value of the drugs that are seized is very small at source. Whilst drugs may be seized with a street value of millions of pounds, this loss is not felt by the producers. The major source of value is contributed by the illegal status of the drugs and the consequent risks taken by those who traffic. But at source, they are cheaply replaced. In summary, therefore, we can say that the last ten or fifteen years have seen a steady increase in the prevalence of drug use and in the number and quantities of illicit substances available to people for illegal use.

What then may we tentatively conclude from these two sets of data? We can say with some certainty that an increase in drug war activity in the UK has not been associated with any decrease in the amount of illegal drug related activity taking place. Indeed, the increase in drug war activity is associated with an increase in all indices of illicit drug use activity. Although it is possible to argue that in the absence of the drug war, current prevalence rates and other drug use statistics might be even higher, we can at best claim that the drug war has possibly slowed down the rate of acceleration in the growth of this problem. However, the cost both in manpower, economic terms and human life occasioned by the war on drugs is difficult to justify on the basis of a possible claim that the drug problem's rate of accelerated increase has in some measurable way been slightly curtailed. Whilst the dynamics of this particular situation are subtle, in lay terms, where a course of activity intended to curtail something is in fact accompanied by an accelerated increase in that activity, one could conclude that the action aimed to curtail the activity is unsuccessful. Even assuming that the drug war has been successful in reducing the rate of increase, one is still entitled to make projections to the future. If current trends continue, we can imagine a situation not too far distant in which the war on drugs becomes a major source of government expenditure, whilst virtually everyone in the population is now an experienced drug user to some level. After all, today's teenagers will constitute the adult population in ten or fifteen years time. In other words simply projecting these two trends into the future does not provide a reassuring picture: it resembles an administration at war with its own people. Reassurance comes only with the assumption that at some point, and for reasons unknown, the drug war suddenly starts to have the effect of reducing the prevalence of drug use. As yet there is no evidence to suggest that this state will ever come about.

CONCLUSION

Let us consider alternative solutions. It takes a rare lack of imagination to persist in the same course of action when all the evidence suggests that this is not particularly effective. Unfortunately data on the consequences of decriminalisation or legalisation of drugs are minimal. There are few satisfactory examples that may be cited in support of the decriminal-isation argument. By virtue of its pragmatic policy towards the drug problem, however, the Netherlands comes under scrutiny. According to one's personal viewpoint, drug policy in the Netherlands is seen either as a brilliant piece of pragmatism which enables that society to cope with the harm that drugs can do in a controlled and acceptable fashion, or alter-natively the Netherlands may be seen as the sick man of Europe whose drug policy threatens to undermine the drug wars being conducted in most other European nations. A recent publication by Junger-Tas *et al.* (eds) (1994) compares data from 13 countries in the western world with respect to a variety of delinquent behaviours. Included in these data are surveys of drug use amongst young people in a number of different nations. We may compare current rates of drug use by aggregating the data from these different studies. Table 12.3 provides a summary of the percentage of representative samples of young people in the countries involved with respect to frequency of their drug use. The data give percentages for those who have ever used drugs and those who have used drugs during the last year.

A number of important points immediately emerge from these data. First, the figures for England and Wales are substantially greater than those for the Netherlands. It should be emphasised that the data from the different countries were collected using identical methods, so the differ-ences in rates cannot be attributed to different methods of data collection. The often quoted argument that due to its process of decriminalisation with respect to cannabis the Netherlands is awash with drugs is simply not supported by these data. What happens is that in the Netherlands visible drug use does indeed take place and is confined to particular areas of Rotterdam, Amsterdam and other towns. In fairness it has to be said that conditions in these 'scene' areas are not particularly appetising. There have also been complaints from residents about the impact of drug use in their areas as a consequence of decriminalisation policy. Whilst

Table 12.3 Prevalence rates (%) for illicit drug use

	Ever used drugs	Used drugs in the last year
Finland	21.9	13.2
England/Wales	34.4	25.9
N. Ireland	24.8	19.9
Netherlands	21.6	15.3
Belgium	13.4	8.2
Germany	14.7	7.0
Switzerland	26.2	20.9
Portugal	19.0	11.3
Spain	21.5	15.4
Italy	8.9	6.3
Greece	12.2	9.1
Midwest USA	26.0	17.3
New Zealand	50.6[a]	63.5

Source: Data abstracted from Junger-Tas *et al.*, 1994

Note: [a] 'ever' items omitted from overseas interviews

accepting these points as valid, it nonetheless remains that prevalence rates in the Netherlands are substantially lower than those in the UK. What is perhaps surprising from these data are the very high rates now being encountered in New Zealand. It remains only to add that during the last decade New Zealand has undergone a change in its philosophy of government, and areas in which community services of various kinds were government funded have been required to become self-financing. New Zealand no longer is the one class society of repute; there are now increasing numbers of people living on voluntary contributions and other non-statutory support of various kinds. It may be that the very high rates of drug use reported in the New Zealand study are related to these deteriorating social conditions.

It is unfortunately the case that conclusions are not inherent in data. It is entirely possible for two people to look at the same data and come up with recommendations for action which are exactly opposite. Science is particularly bad at answering questions that imply an 'ought'. For example, whilst physicists may unravel the secrets of nuclear fission, the practical problems of whether one should build nuclear power stations or nuclear weapons remain unaddressed by the scientific data. These merely specify the different courses of action that are possible. Consequently in the present circumstances, conclusions from data of the above kinds are matters for discussion. That having been said, it is the firm opinion of the writer that only one of the above philosophies for dealing with drug problems offers any hope for the future. That option involves the progressive decriminalisation of drugs and the progressive implementation of strategies of harm reduction for those people whose drug use creates problems at a personal, family or social level.

REFERENCES

Addiction Research (1994) *Special Issue. Cocaine in the community: International perspectives*, Vol. 2, No. 1, Switzerland: Harwood Academic Publishers.

Coggans, N., Shewan, D., Henderson, M., and Davies, J. B. (1991) *National Evaluation of Drug Education in Scotland: ISDD Research Monograph Four*, London: Institute for the Study of Drug Dependence.

Davies, J. B. and Coggans, N. (1991) *The Facts about Adolescent Drug Abuse*, London: Cassell.

Doll, R., Peto, R., Hall, E., Wheatly, K. and Gray, R. (1994) 'Mortality in relation to consumption of alcohol: 13 years' observations of British male doctors', *British Medical Journal* 309: 911–18.

Haw, S. (1989) 'The sentencing of drug offenders in Scottish Courts', Report to SHHD Criminology and Law Research Group, SHHD Library.

Hawkins, J. D., Catalano, F. and Millar, J. Y. (1992) 'Risk and protective factors for alcohol and other drug problems in adolescence and early childhood: implications for substance abuse prevention', *Psychological Bulletin* 112, 1: 64–105.

Henderson, M. M., Coggans, N. and Davies, J. B. (1993) *Evaluation of Health and HIV/AIDS Education*, Commissioned and published by Argyll and Clyde Health Board (Health Promotion Department).

Junger-Tas, J., Terlouw, G. J., Klein, M. W. (eds) (1994) *Delinquent Behaviour among Young People in the Western World: First Results of the International Self-report Delinquency Study*, Amsterdam/New York: Kluger Publications.

Leuw, E. and Haen Marshall, I. (eds) (1994) *Between Prohibition and Legislation: The Dutch Experiment in Drug Policy*, Amsterdam: Kluger Publications.

McAleese, K. (1994) 'Student drugs survey', *Strathclyde Telegraph* 3, 35: 6–8.

McMurran, M. (1994) *The Psychology of Addiction*, London: Taylor & Francis.

Newcombe, R., Measham, F. and Parker, H. J. (1994) 'The normalisation of recreational drug use amongst young people in North West England', *British Journal of Sociology* 45: 307–32.

Parker, H. J. and Measham, F. (1994) 'Pick 'n' mix: patterns of illicit drug use amongst 1990's adolescents', *Drugs: Education Prevention Policy* 1, 1: 5–14.

Plant, M. A., Peck, D. and Samuel, E. (1985) *Alcohol, Drugs and School Leavers*, London: Tavistock.

Report of the Surgeon General (1989) *The Health Consequences of Smoking: Nicotine Addicton*, Rockville: US Department of Health and Human Resources.

Royal College of Psychiatrists (1987) *Drug Scenes*, London: Gaskell.

Swadi, H. (1988) 'Drug and substance use among 3,333 London adolescents', *British Journal of Addiction*, 83: 935–42.

Szasz, T. S. (1985) *Ceremonial Chemistry: The Ritual Persecution of Drugs, Addicts and Pushers*, Revised Edition, Holmes Beach: Learning Publications Inc.

Chapter 13

Drug abuse: the issue of prevention

John B. Davies

In the light of the previous chapter, it will be apparent that the issue of prevention presents a number of problems. If one takes the view that a future may be envisaged within which nobody uses any illicit substances, and that such a state is both feasible and achievable, the issue of prevention centres around those policies and strategies necessary to eliminate drug use from our midst. On the other hand if an approach is taken that, like it or not, the use of illicit mind-altering substances is here to stay and has to be lived with, then different issues arise. A central one is 'How do we prevent people who indulge in the use of illicit drugs from coming to harm?' and the related question 'How do we minimise the dangers and harm that will surely occur to a small percentage of those who do choose to take part in these activities?' In other words, before deciding on a prevention strategy one has to consider in some detail the thorny question 'Prevention of what?'.

Whichever route one wishes to take, either the prevention of drug use *per se* or the prevention of harm arising from such activity, education is seen by most as the key to progress. The reason why people prefer the educational route is perhaps because it involves minimal change and minimal inconvenience for the rest of society as a whole, rather than because education has been shown to be the most effective strategy. Despite the fact that drug use tends to be at its most ugly in areas of inner city urban decay and deprivation, the belief that education will solve the problems appears to remove from society at large any requirement to change the physical and social world within which drug use frequently manifests itself. By choosing education as a central preventative measure, we assume that progress can be made without any major readjustments to the social and economic world in which we live. It goes without saying, however, that whilst education plays a pivotal role in preparing young people of all ages and social classes for the world in which they are going to live, it is unlikely to solve the problems of drug abuse unless supported by concrete changes to social policy in other areas. Drug education has a crucial role but is unlikely to be sufficient to the task unless supported in other ways.

It appears, however, that many people believe drug education by itself will be quite sufficient and that there is a large body of evidence indicating that 'it works'. It may come as a surprise, therefore, to learn that despite the large amount of money spent on drug and related education, and the increasing sophistication of the approaches being used (particularly in schools) there is a shortage of clear-cut information indicating that specific educational campaigns have produced identifiable reductions in substance use. A much cited study in the US by Kinder *et al.* (1980), admittedly now slightly out of date, sparked off the argument in a review of over one hundred drug education programmes. The majority of these had no impact on reported levels of substance use amongst the targeted groups. A smaller proportion had some slight positive effect but a number actually had a small but measurable negative effect. A rough and ready conclusion from this and similar studies might be that whilst occasionally a programme is seen to produce lower reports of drug use amongst children, there are also a disturbing number of studies which show exactly the opposite; and a majority of studies which fail to show any difference either way. If 'drug stopping' is the aim, therefore, there is surprisingly little evidence that education is effective; and that statement remains broadly as true today as it was in 1980.

However, drug education campaigns in the UK have moved on from the days of Kinder *et al.* Progress has been made not so much in terms of efficacy in respect of reducing levels of drug use, as in regard to the philosophy of providing drug education in the first place. The 'Life Skills' approach to drug education (to be discussed later) is generally more concerned with preparing youngsters to deal with the problems of drug use that they may encounter, less with the goal of stamping out drug use *per se*. Consequently evaluations of drug education have drifted away from the hard-nosed, probably unattainable goal of reducing or eliminating drug use to the goals of ensuring that youngsters are aware of the facts with respect to drugs, injecting, AIDS/HIV and so forth and have acquired the life skills to enable them to navigate their way about a drug-using world, regardless of whether they decide to use or not. The goals of drug education have thus subtly changed.

FEAR AROUSAL

Different approaches have been used towards drug education in the past. Currently the dialectical approach based on life skills is favoured amongst educationists themselves. However, amongst the lay public and in government, traditional approaches whose main virtue is that they make the deliverer of the education feel righteous, are still preferred. Foremost amongst these is the technique of *fear arousal*, an approach which seeks to put young people off using drugs by showing catastrophic, but usually exaggerated, consequences. Research by Finnigan (1988) showed that whilst drug users themselves were more open to persuasion by messages that stressed the damaging social consequences of their drug use on their families and children, members of the lay public nonetheless felt that the best drug education messages were those based on a technique of arousing fear about illness and death of the user.

Fear arousal is based on the idea that people can be frightened out of their bad habits. Such campaigns therefore centre around visual images of death and disaster and verbal labels like 'the effects can last forever'. The technique of fear arousal has been much researched in the literature but remains little understood by the public at large. A general feeling amongst the lay public and many politicians is that this approach is the best way forward. However, amongst educators there is a tendency to view fear arousal, with some justification, as ineffective. In fact the truth lies somewhere between the two. Excellent review articles have been produced on the topic, (e.g. Sutton, 1982). It is not the case that fear arousal is a good way of approaching problems such as drug misuse, but neither is it the case that fear arousal has no application at all. It depends, amongst other things, on the level of knowledge and familiarity of the subject matter in the target population. However, a number of workers have found fear arousal in the context of drug education campaigns to be ineffective and alienating (Le Dain, 1970, Smart and Fejer, 1974). It is interesting to note that the government's own advisory body, the Advisory Council on the Misuse of Drugs (ACMD) took the view in their report on prevention in 1984 that 'Drug education should not concentrate solely on factual information about drug misuse, even less present such information in a way that is intended to shock or scare'.

Where an activity or an object is unfamiliar and strange, people can sometimes be 'inoculated' ('stopping them starting') by means of fear arousal techniques, because they have no store of everyday or mundane experience with which to compare the fear arousal message. In such circumstances many members of a target audience are likely to accept the message at face value. We have seen, however, that amongst teenagers, drug use runs at a level of between 30 per cent and 40 per cent in the UK. This means that almost half of youngsters will have some personal experience of use of illicit drugs. Virtually all of them, however, will have at least second-hand experience of illicit drugs in the form of friends or acquaintances who have used drugs, and who are in most cases still attending school and functioning normally. The fear arousal message at best is ineffective for behaviour change because the fear aroused is seen to be quite disproportionate to the actual level of damage experienced or observed. It is not possible to frighten people out of things that they do with some regularity and which are observed to have few long-term consequences. Moreover, a negative goal may be achieved in these circumstances. Exaggerated, biased and (not to put too fine a point on it) untruthful messages that underlie much fear arousing drug education discredit the *source* of the information. They also discredit the source not merely with respect to drug education but with respect to other topics where the information may be less biased, often by undermining the credibility of health and social education sources on a broader front.

INFORMATION

If we cannot frighten youngsters out of their drug use, maybe another approach is desirable. The information-based approach has been much publicised. According to this, youngsters require factual information about risky activities on the basis of which to make rational decisions about their own behaviour. This liberal and democratic model, however, is underlaid by some assumptions. It is assumed in some quarters that people will only use drugs as long as they are unaware of information about the consequences. This is simply not the case. Generally speaking people do not take part in risky activities simply because they are un- aware of the consequences of such behaviour. Rock climbers are well aware of the consequences of falling. Parachutists and sky divers are well aware of the consequences of the parachute failing to open, and so on. In a similar way it is probably wrong to characterise the majority of drug use, sexual behaviour or other adolescent problem behaviours as deriving solely from a lack of information. With respect to drugs, it is often claimed by drug workers that the children know rather more than their parents and teachers.

The second assumption behind certain information-based approaches is slightly more hypocritical. The information is provided ostensibly so that youngsters will be able to make 'informed' decisions. However, there is a strong suspicion that one of these decisions is a 'right' decision whilst the other is a 'wrong' decision. Mixing up the information-based approach with clear indications that one type of decision is better than another is a sure way to invalidate this kind of education. Interviews with children from our own studies suggest that they are well aware when they are being 'got at' which can be expected to provoke a reaction entirely opposite from that required. An extensive review by Schaps *et al.* (1981) revealed the limitations of the information-based approach; and also showed, disturbingly, that such an approach might be associated with outcomes in some instances opposite to those intended.

HARM REDUCTION

A radical approach to drug education involves the problematic and con- tentious issue of harm reduction. Harm reduction has a number of faces and there may be internal logical and definitional problems with the concept (Strang, 1993). Its specific aim is to provide information and services for those who do use drugs and who may encounter problems by virtue of that drug use. The aim is neither to stop nor reduce drug use on a broad front, but to minimise the damage caused to that smaller number of people who use drugs unwisely and experience problems as a result. Harm reduction might manifest itself in unpredictable and often disturbing ways. On the one hand it might involve providing information within a clinic about the need to use clean, sterilised needles in the interests of avoiding AIDS and HIV. At the other extreme it might involve such interventions as the widespread dissemination of the notorious 'Chill-Out' leaflet that circulated Liverpool discotheques and night spots during 1990. This leaflet gave explicit directions to ecstasy users about how to take the drugs, the quantities which should be taken and the ways of avoiding negative side effects. The pamphlet caused outrage amongst the conservative press and the broader cross-section of 'right thinking' individuals. In a similar vein a number of angry and outraged parents attended a conference in Glasgow, where they made their views forcefully known concerning the distribution by a local agency of harm reduction literature to children aged between 11 and 14 years in a number of schools in deprived areas of the city. These parents saw this type of intervention as inappropriate, and as in effect providing 'how to do it' information for youngsters who, arguably, were better off without that knowledge.

Finally, perhaps one of the more contentious recent publications is the 110 page *Anabolic Reference Guide* now running to a fifth underground edition, the most recent of which was published in 1991. This comprehensive work gives specific guidance to athletes on how to 'cycle' their steroid use so as to avoid negative health consequences, whilst improving their performance; and also how to manage their drug use in such a way as to avoid detection. The guide is well referenced and is a work of some medical scholarship. Its ethical status, however is very much a matter of personal view. It certainly constitutes an authoritative and thoroughgoing contribution to harm reduction education, though we might argue about whose harm is being reduced, and at what cost.

THE PROBLEMS OF TARGET GROUPS AND FALSE POSITIVES

Ethical debates cannot be resolved by science. In 1739, Hume showed that statements about what we 'ought' to do cannot be derived from descriptions of what is. However, the problems arising from various approaches to drug use may nonetheless be addressed so as to inform the debate at a pragmatic, if not at an ethical, level. Hence, the approach of these two chapters has been that only pragmatic solutions are likely to offer any long-term beneficial consequences to society and that the pursuit of ethical truths with respect to the misuse of illicit drugs is a wild goose chase.

Central to issues around drug education is the problem of false positives, a term derived in the first instance from the science of 'decision theory', although the basic philosophy applies in a number of other areas including screening tests, inoculation against disease and the provision of drug education. In the area of drug education we may conceptualise the 'false positive' problem in terms of a two by two matrix. The two by two matrix is derived from considering the conjunction of a particular intervention and its appropriateness for a particular target audience. At risk of over-simplifying what happens in the real world we may construct our two by two matrix as shown in Figure 13.1.

First let us suppose we have a drug education package intended to stop users from using ('starting them stopping'). The choice is whether to use the package or not. Secondly let us suppose that we have just two target groups, those who use drugs and those who do not. Whilst admitting the highly over-simplified picture of the world presented by the above matrix, formulating the problem in this way leads to some interesting implications. Given a choice of (1) whether to provide this particular drug education or not, and (2) a target group which uses drugs or which does not, breaks the issue down into four cells. They are as follows: first, we may imagine a group of drug users who could receive drug education. This represents the state of affairs in the top left hand box and in decision theory parlance the numbers in this box would be termed 'hits', that is, the education 'hits' this number of appropriate 'target' persons. Second, we have a group of non-users who have not used drugs and who have possibly never considered doing so. If such a group receives no drug education, the state of affairs would be represented by the box in the lower right corner of the matrix, termed 'correct negatives'. Our drug education pack would be inappropriate for this group, given its aim (i.e. 'starting them stopping'). The two remaining boxes represent 'misses'

	Users	Non-users
Receive 'stopping' education	Hits	False positives
Do not receive 'stopping' education	Misses	Correct negatives

Figure 13.1 Outcome matrix for an education initiative aimed at stopping drug use.

and 'false positives'. In the upper right box, we have a group of users, that is, a potential target group, who for whatever reason, fails to receive any drug education. The numbers in this box would be termed 'misses'. The final box in the lower left hand corner is the most important. This is a group who have not used drugs, who nonetheless receive drug education intended to stop use. This is the 'false positive' rate, important because it represents a number of individuals whose interest in drugs and their use is potentially (or actually) aroused by the education itself.

Consideration of the matrix centres on the ratio of 'hits' to 'false positives'. Where the numbers of a potential target audience in the general population are small, (i.e. there are relatively few users), the chance exists that in return for delivering an appropriate message to users, a greater degree of harm is done by extending the message to a larger number of non-users who thereby constitute a high 'false positive' risk. On the other hand, if the number of users in a population is large and the number of non-users is small, then the trade off between 'hits' and 'false positives' is probably worthwhile. In return for arousing an interest that was not there before in a small number of people, we convey an appropriate message to a larger subsection who comprise an appropriate target group.

At the present time we have seen that drug use amongst youngsters runs at the level of some 30 to 40 per cent. Given this level of activity and interest, drug education of whatever type becomes more justifiable. Furthermore, as the number of users in the population increases, so education becomes *more* justifiable although not necessarily increasingly effective. It can be argued (but not proved), that a contributor to the current high levels of use has been the unwarranted level of concern and attention attracted by drug misuse during the late 1960s and early 1970s at which times the prevalence of drug use amongst young people was lower, whilst the level of concern was almost the same as it is today. Taking an inappropriately 'over the top' approach to drug education campaigns and disseminating messages through the mass media at times when prevalence of drug use in a population is low may actually stimulate the growth of a drug problem in that population, by virtue of the fact that the ratio of false positives to hits is very high. Whatever the truth of this speculation, we now live in a world where drug education is increasingly necessary and where prevalence of use makes drug education progressively more justifiable. With respect to earlier endeavours, we might contemplate the possibility that colourful drug campaigns were successful in the UK and USA in helping to win elections, but did little to help the drug problem.

Obviously, the implications of the decision theory analogy vary for different kinds of education. Thus, education aimed at primary prevention ('stopping them starting') would in principle target the non-drug using sections of the population. On the other hand, education directed towards 'starting them stopping' would be targeted at the using section of the population. Since the proportions of users and non-users vary according to the age of the target population, and since also these relative proportions change reciprocally over time, a cost/benefit analysis of either of these approaches has to take such age and time trends into account. For example, the primary prevention message aimed at an age group where drug users are in a majority at a given point in time will be largely a waste of resources. By contrast a secondary prevention message used with an age group amongst whom drug use prevalence is low, or a broader population within which drug users are in a minority, runs the risk of arousing more interest, whilst being of direct relevance to only a few people.

These kinds of targeting problems are possibly most acute with respect to the harm reduction approach in so far as part of its philosophy involves giving specific instructions about how to use drugs safely. This is a message which may perhaps be more harmful than any other if targeted where the false positives are high. For this reason there are serious questions to be asked about the general applicability of a harm reduction approach at the population level. It has been advocated in some circles that even amongst primary school children harm reduction is now appropriate because *some* children of below the age of ten are using drugs. To adopt a broad scale harm reduction approach with this age group is thus to make the phenomenon of child drug use more salient amongst this group of children as a whole. Accordingly the false positive rate will be high and we may thus expect an increase in awareness and interest in this younger age group as a consequence of such harm reduction education. This may or may not be a step in the right direction.

On the other hand, the impact of the harm reduction approach is entirely justified where the target audience consists largely of people to whom the harm reduction message is appropriate. For example, the 'Chill-Out' leaflet targeted at youngsters attending raves in Liverpool, mentioned above, can only be seen as a good thing in those circumstances. It may be the case that government ministers have only just discovered that people go to raves in order to get drugs; however, this has widely been known both amongst ravers and drug workers for some years. The 'Chill-Out' leaflet is therefore an example of well targeted harm-reduction education of a kind which will achieve maximum hits and minimise false positives, providing this is targeted in the way described. Similarly it may be expected that the *Anabolic Reference Guide* would be mainly of interest to athletes using drugs in order to enhance their performance. Provided that is the target group which the guide reaches, rather more benefit than harm may be achieved. On the other hand where these kinds of harm minimisation approaches are not appropriately targeted, the false positive rate will be high and may cancel out any benefit, or worse.

The logic of targeting and the way this interacts with the possible costs and benefits of particular educational initiatives is thus easy to see. However, in a sense we have swapped the ethical issues about whether it is morally right or wrong to use drugs for a purely pragmatic approach; and in the process we have now merely shifted the ethical debate to that of targeting groups. To view groups of teenagers using illicit drugs at a disco as a target group does not, in the opinion of the author, breach any strong ethical considerations, though some people would argue that parental consent should be necessary for any interventions of this kind before any such steps would taken, i.e. the dissemination of the 'Chill-Out' leaflet. But given the potential dangers of the unwise use of illicit drugs the relationship between drug use and sexual behaviour, and thereby the link between drug use and HIV/AIDS, it is important that those directly involved in the front line, (i.e. the regular users) acquire the information that is necessary to enable them to navigate these difficult waters. Given the risk of AIDS and HIV this is arguably a more important consideration than keeping parents happy.

TARGETING THOSE AT RISK

However, it is possible to envisage situations in which such common-sense views of 'right' and 'wrong' do not so readily emerge. In recent literature a number of risk and preventive factors with respect to drug use amongst young people have been identified, (e.g. Hawkins *et al.*, 1992). These data have been derived largely from studies of young people, in which a number of factors have been identified which discriminate users from non-users. It is thus in principle possible to identify groups of youngsters who have higher scores on those 'risk factors' and who may therefore be said to be groups *most at risk* of either illicit drug use or experiencing drug problems. Regardless of the methodological adequacy of some of these researches, the logic of such targeting (even if the studies were impeccable) remains somewhat problematic. The idea of targeting particular sub-groups of youngsters as being at risk from the problems of drug abuse, at a time before any such abuse (or indeed even any use) has taken place raises the most taxing ethical dilemmas, central to which are the problems of labelling and self-fulfilling prophecies. Whilst it is clear that many youngsters using drugs show a full constellation of risk factors, it is also the case that there are also many youngsters with a 'full set' of risk factors who do not use drugs, or who use drugs occasionally, in a non-problematic fashion. Any targeting that took place on the basis of risk factors would necessarily include numbers of youngsters who, left to their own devices would subsequently not develop drug problems, or even any drug use, despite their 'at risk' status. The problem arises as a consequence of the earlier discussions of false positives and the appropriateness of education to particular groups. There are obviously logical advantages in being able to target education at those groups who are most at risk for the activity in question. However, taking this argument to a finer level reveals an even more stark ethical dilemma than drug use itself, namely the problem of labelling large sections of the population at risk for a particular activity, treating them as though they were all the same, and giving them specific educational materials based on that labelling exercise.

SUMMARY

There is no doubt of the advantages of specifically engineered education messages, be they fear arousal, harm reduction, information, or whatever, specifically and appropriately targeted at groups to whom they are appropriate. One might expect in such circumstances to see more direct and tangible evidence of the effect of health education. But the ethical dilemmas raised are frightening. Consequently, education seems to proceed on the basis of hope for the most part, providing messages for general consumption which fail to grasp central issues about whether to use or not to use and which generally fall somewhere in the no-man's-land between fear arousal and information provision.

The most recent and hopeful development in the area of education has been the life skills approach which in a sense circumnavigates some of these problems by attempting to shape young people's perceptions of the world and of each other in helpful ways that will improve self-efficacy, confidence, social skills and so forth but only targets the specific issue of drug use in a tangential way.

CONCLUSIONS

A great deal of energy and effort has been invested over the last two decades in the production of drug education packages primarily aimed at youngsters of school age. It is worth noting in passing that the section of the population that experiences the most difficult problems with drug abuse is not actually this age group. Nonetheless they are the ones most frequently targeted. On a positive note it must be said that in an increasingly complex world where drugs and alcohol are increasingly available some preparation by way of education is necessary to enable youngsters to cope with these difficult pressures. It must also be said that some of the packages that have been produced are elegant, creative and innovative and contrast with some of the more stereotyped fear and information-based approaches that characterised early endeavours.

Whilst the life skills and other reflexive methods seem to provide youngsters with the most involving and positive forms of educational experience, it remains to be said that evidence indicating that education about drugs produces any measurable reduction in use is very hard to find. Indeed data covering the last fifteen years tend to show increases in consumption for most age groups across the board despite increases in the amount of education being made available. Whilst fully acknowledging the place of such education within the school and the broader social curriculum, a realistic appraisal must lead to the conclusion that solutions to the problems of drug use, particularly amongst young people, are unlikely to be found via the educational route alone. It seems unlikely that anyone will come up with the drug education package that works for everyone at all times and in all circumstances.

The problems of drug use are closely tied to a number of characteristics of the social and economic world in which we live. Within that world large numbers of people of all ages find positive effects from taking illicit drugs in full knowledge that this is a dangerous activity which may have serious consequences for some of them. The same is true for licit drugs. The data suggest, however, that the numbers who experience serious consequences from illicit drug use are rather small, though they are rising. Consequently messages based on fear cannot succeed since the activity is familiar personally to roughly half the target audience and at second hand to most of it.

Longer term solutions to the problems of drugs require a re-appraisal of the kind of world in which we all live and the kinds of things that people find rewarding or satisfying within that society. In our present post-enlightenment society we pursue a 'gesellschaft' existence (Hollinger, 1994). A 'gesellschaft' society is basically a society of strangers based on technology and science. The demands of production and trade require the break up of smaller family units and within such a system a return to established and enduring cultural and family values relating to 'right' and 'wrong' is probably impossible. In such a setting we may expect a reduction in the consensus about those kinds of behaviours which may or may not be tolerated, and disagreements about what is or is not acceptable. That is the price we pay for living in an open and flexible society that prizes individual freedom. Also within that society the proliferation of different types of substances which change the operation of the mind and their availability through legal and illegal routes to large sections of the population seems an inevitable development. In such a setting education requires to be as much about preparing people for that world as about stopping them from doing 'bad' things.

Within such a social context the notion of harm reduction is bound progressively to come to the fore, and be seen as appropriate in more and more settings. We have seen how there are possibilities for targeting particular sections of the population with messages that are most appropriate to their needs and behaviour, and harm reduction clearly has an important role, along with other approaches. We have also seen how the problems of targeting create the associated problems of false positives and promote discussion about the costs and benefits of a particular approach. Whilst at the present time the government and media persist in straightforward, if misguided, anti-drug messages, there is at the other extreme an evangelical fringe that appears to favour harm reduction for all. Under this second heading, the fact that some youngsters in primary school dabble with drugs becomes a banner under which drug education for all children within that age group is now being advocated. In fact if progress is to be assured, a detailed and informed discussion of the costs and benefits of targeting particular groups with particular types of message is now required, as opposed to the general dissemination of 'don't do it' messages to youngsters, many of whom do it already; or on the other hand, a harm reduction 'free for all'.

REFERENCES

Advisory Council on the Misuse of Drugs (1984) *Prevention*, London: HMSO.

Finnigan, F. (1988) 'Stereotyping in addiction: an application of the Fishbein-Ajzen theory to heroin using behaviour', Ph.D. thesis, University of Strathclyde Library.

Hawkins, J. D., Catalano, R. F. and Miller, J. Y. (1992) 'Risk and protective factors for alcohol and other drug problems in adolescence and early adulthood: implications for substance use prevention', *Psychological Bulletin* 112, 1: 64–105.

Hollinger, R. (1994) *Postmodernism and the Social Sciences: A Thematic Approach*, London: Sage.

Hume, D. (1739) *A Treatise on Human Nature* (originally published 1739) L. A. Selby-Bigge (ed.) (1888) Oxford: Oxford University Press.

Kinder, B. N., Pape, N. E. and Walfish, S. (1980) 'Drug and alcohol education programs: a review of outcome studies', *International Journal of the Addictions*, 15: 1035–54.

Le Dain, G. (1970) *Interim Report of the Commission of Inquiry into the Non-medical Use of Drugs*, Ottawa: Information Canada.

Schaps, E., Di Bartolo, R., Moskowitz, J. M., Palley, C. and Chugrins, S. (1981) 'A review of 127 drug abuse prevention program evaluations', *Journal of Drug Issues*, 11: 17–44.

Smart, R. G. and Fejer, D. (1974) 'The effects of high and low fear arousal messages about drugs', *Journal of Drug Education*, 4: 225–35.

Strang, J. (1993) 'Drug use and harm reduction: responding to the challenge', in N. Heather, A. Wodak, E. Nadelman and P. O'Hare (eds), *Harm Reduction: from Faith to Science*, London: Wurr Publishers.

Sutton, S. R. (1982) 'Fear-arousing communications: a critical examination of theory and research', in J. R. Eiser, (ed.) *Social Psychology and Behavioural Medicine*, Chichester: Wiley.

Index